I0429481

IT'S NOT THE COOKIE, IT'S THE BAG:

An Easy-To-Follow Guide for Weight Loss Success

Maxwell Ivey Jr.

It's Not the Cookie, It's the Bag: An Easy-to-Follow Guide for Weight Loss Success

Copyright © 2016 by Maxwell Ivey Jr.
All rights reserved.

ISBN-13: 978-1532713231

No part of this book may be reproduced in any form or by any means electronically or otherwise, unless permission has been granted by the author, with the exception of brief excerpts for review purposes.

Cover creation and formatting for printing by Brenda from www.coversbydesign.net

Layout, formatting, and editing courtesy of Lorraine Reguly from www.wordingwell.com

Dedication

This book is dedicated to anyone who wants to make healthier decisions and become the person you want to be... the person you were meant to be... the person you *deserve* to be.

Table of Contents

Introduction

Hello. My name is Max, and I like to write as though I am talking to my best friend.

I am an almost totally blind gentleman from Conroe, Texas, which is near Houston, in the United States of America. I'm currently 50 years old. I am 6'4", weigh 250 pounds, and am in the best physical health of my life.

Not only am I an author, I am a successful blogger, coach, and entrepreneur. I own two businesses and I have a wealth of supportive friends, both online and off.

However, it wasn't always this way.

After the early death of my father in 2003, my brothers and I were unable to keep the family-owned business going. We had operated a traveling carnival, like many of our relatives had done—and are still doing. After we went out of business, we had to go to work with my uncle's carnival. We had competed with his family for bookings, so this made the feeling of failure that much worse.

My health declined and I was on my way to an early death. I had high blood pressure. I took a variety of medications. I was morbidly obese. I was depressed. I was also not sure where I was going in life.

I barely had the energy or passion to do much more than get out of bed each morning. I was sleeping on the floor of a travel trailer at the time.

Basically, *I was a mess.*

I started my transformation by getting healthy.

I went from being a miserable, 512-pound man to a happy guy who now weighs 250 pounds. I had gastric surgery to help me lose the weight, but I had to lose weight first in order to get the surgery.

In this book, I will share the secrets of my weight loss. I will teach you how you can achieve the same results I did. The best part? You do not have to have gastric surgery in order to see results!

Are you ready? Good. Let's dive in, and start at the beginning of my journey, a journey I continue to take each day; a journey to happiness that you can follow, too.

Starting Your Transformation

I'm going to begin by telling you a bit about what I was feeling on October 2nd, 2012, when I showed up at the hospital to have my gastric surgery.

I have been fat all my life. When I was young, people used words like *husky* and *chunky*, but let's face it—I have always been overweight. I grew up in a large family of carnival owners. At that time, the industry was more heavy equipment than high-tech, so it made sense for show owners to have large families of strapping young men.

This was fine when I was young, but not as great as I got older. And when the death of my father resulted in our family's carnival going out of business, my health got even worse.

Over the years, I have tried to lose weight many times. I didn't try any of the really crazy diets; I always used a variation of healthier eating and exercise. This would work for short periods but would usually fall by the wayside once we started traveling for our work.

So, after trying and failing *and trying and failing*, my primary care doctor asked me to attend a seminar on weight loss surgeries. I agreed to go and listen. She had just put me on Metformin, a drug for diabetics.

I went to the seminar, and my mind was opened to the possibility of surgery to help me lose weight. The presenters convinced me that the procedure was just the first step in a long line of steps that I would need to take for this to work out well—for me to have a healthier life. So, when I went into surgery that morning I wasn't afraid. I wasn't afraid of the surgery because I had gotten to know the surgeon and his staff so well that I trusted them. More importantly, I wasn't worried about not losing the weight because of all the tools and techniques I had learned while preparing to have the surgery.

That's why I decided to write this book. I know not everyone is a good candidate for surgery. And I learned a lot of real-life lessons and techniques that can be applied to YOU and your life, whether you need to lose 10 pounds or 300.

I won't say that preparing for the procedure was easy, or that the first few months after having it weren't hard, but I was confident that this time I would succeed. I was at peace with the whole idea of changing my perspective of who I am. Going from over

500 pounds down to 250 means a big change in how you see yourself even if you can't see yourself. (Wink, wink!)

Now, I want to tell you a bit about myself and this journey I've been on.

As I mentioned in the introduction, I am a totally blind gentleman from Conroe, Texas, who lost over 250 pounds.

I did it by having gastric surgery, changing my diet, getting regular exercise, and tapping into the power of prayer, meditation, and a positive attitude.

I'm currently in the best shape of my life and very happy with my body. I am able to maintain my weight without a major struggle. I have successfully navigated several Thanksgiving and Christmas holiday seasons. I have even taken short trips without it affecting my health.

At the time of this writing, the 2015 Christmas holidays have just ended. All those ads on television for diets, exercise equipment, fitness centers, and weight loss plans got me to thinking. I thought maybe people would benefit from what I learned as I prepared for having the surgery. I thought I could also discuss some of the adjustments I have made now that I am living with my weight loss several years after having the surgery.

The first thing I learned was that having a gastric procedure was not like waving a magic wand and solving all of my weight problems. Surgery is just a tool to make it easier for you to succeed. You still have to put in the work and make the effort to change your lifestyle.

The second thing that I learned was that having an operation wasn't admitting I was a failure. I am not so weak or so lacking in willpower that I can't lose the weight and keep it off. And having the procedure didn't make me a quitter. In fact, only about fifty percent of people who have weight loss surgery will lose eighty to ninety percent of the weight they need to lose.

In order to get the maximum benefit from the surgery, you have to be willing to make many difficult changes in your life. I can honestly say that I am not the same person today that I was almost four years ago. They say that if one spouse gets healthy, and the other does not, there is a high probability that a divorce will result. I can believe this because weight loss does, indeed, affect your personality.

For people like me that needed to lose hundreds of pounds, it requires learning to see yourself in a whole new way.

When it comes to food, my attitudes are much different now. Thanks to the surgery, I get full faster than I did before, and because of what I learned from the dietitians and nutritionists, I now make much better food choices.

But I am not perfect. I still have days where I will eat a little too much or will have something that I know isn't good for me. Even our instructors admitted to doing this! There are days when I don't feel like exercising, or life interferes with my work-out time. This just means I have to start over again the next day, and so will you.

Once you lose weight, if you notice yourself starting to put back on a pound or two, you will remind yourself of what got you to the body you wanted. You will decide that you don't want to waste all that hard work you put in, and then you go back to what works.

I will tell you that it's not always easy. It does take some getting used to. Losing weight requires thought, careful planning, and some determination. But I'll help you with that! Also, don't think that I'm going to try to talk you into having some sort of surgery or that my suggestions will only work if you have a huge amount of weight to lose. I know having gastric surgery isn't required by most people and isn't effective unless that person wants to make real changes in their life.

Many of the ideas included in this book came to me during the time leading up to having the surgery. It took six months before my insurance company would approve me to have the operation. In that time, I lost 81 pounds. (I weighed 512 pounds on February 14th, 2012, when I had my first official weigh-in. I was down to 431 pounds by the time I had my surgery on October 2nd, 2012.)

The same methods I have used will be helpful to you whether you need to lose a lot of weight or are just needing help losing that "extra ten pounds."

At this point, I should mention that I don't have any formal training in the areas of fitness or nutrition. I don't have any degrees or certifications.

I am sharing what I learned from my instructors along with my personal take on how these changes can be more easily integrated into a real, every-day, normal, hectic life.

My suggestions may not work for you exactly as how they worked for me, but they should give you new ideas about how you can make changes to your life to achieve your goals.

My experiences should help you be more creative at finding ways of becoming healthier and staying healthier. I am hopeful that you can use my example to be more loving towards yourself and accepting of your body. And most of all, I'm hoping that, after hearing that I have done it, you will decide you can and will do it for yourself.

I believe in a total body approach to success, regardless of your goal. I firmly believe that you have to get healthy physically, mentally, emotionally, and spiritually before you can achieve your heart's desires and other long-term goals. In fact, I didn't even realize I wanted to do most of the things I now do until after I started down the path towards better physical well-being.

Making positive changes will have a snowball effect on you.

The more steps you take, the more you will *want* to take. The more progress you make, the more areas of your life that you will see opportunities in.

Since I started my journey, I have gone from a failed carnival owner to a successful amusement equipment broker. I went from being morbidly obese and taking seven different prescriptions to being completely free of prescription medicines and being at the best weight in my life. I have become a respected blogger, coach, and self-published author. I have recorded audios, videos, and have become a prolific guest of podcasts and radio shows. I am going to be sharing my message of taking action and overcoming your obstacles at live events later this year.

And who knows what else is in my future!

This is what I meant about how your life will open up with many new opportunities and challenges as you start getting in better shape. This is because you will start to see new opportunities *everywhere*.

When I went to the classes prior to my surgery, they told us to start looking for a hobby or a new venture. They said this was because eventually we would have so much more energy and we would need an outlet for it.

I didn't believe them one hundred percent at the time, but I believe them now!

What would you be doing differently right now if you were in better health to accomplish it? Would you be starting a new business, finding a new romance, taking up a new hobby, be planning an amazing trip, or going back to school?

Whatever your goal is, just remember that having the belief in yourself to go after it is another benefit of losing weight and keeping it off.

Success in one area of your life will lead to success in all the others. Now, let's get started!

How to Keep a Proper Food Journal

If you have been trying unsuccessfully to lose weight for a long time, then you must have, at some point, heard about keeping a food journal.

When I started preparing to have the surgery, our instructors encouraged us to keep one, too. I had done so a few times before, so I decided not to. I wasn't being rebellious. I just knew that it wouldn't work for me.

The reason for this is because a food journal is designed to help you see where you are making your mistakes. The purpose is to figure out what you are eating, when you eat it, and, most importantly, *why you are eating*.

Well, I knew what my problem was. I was eating what appeared to be a relatively healthy diet, but I was not losing any weight.

I had attended the seminar and decided that making my stomach smaller and changing my body's idea of how much I could eat was the only way to solve my problem permanently. I didn't believe this prior to attending the presentation on what gastric surgery is and isn't, so I didn't keep a food journal.

19

Most of us we know what our problem areas are. We know who or what generally triggers us to eat. We know what foods to avoid. The difficulty comes from implementing what we learned about ourselves by keeping a food journal.

If you are going to keep a food journal, here are some pointers on how to do it in a manner that will give you some real results.

First, *don't* share your journal with anyone other than a doctor or therapist. Sharing these details with anyone else is not healthy.

This is because *when you share, you compare*. You worry about what others will think of what you had for lunch that day. Even with our spouses or best friends, we are tempted to lie. We will change the big juicy cheeseburger to a half a tuna sandwich on whole wheat bread with no mayonnaise. We will say we ate three cookies when really it was six, or twelve, or more. We will say we didn't have any chips when there is half a bag gone.

The same thing applies to exercise. You'll say you walked two miles when all you did was put on your shoes and think about walking.

When you know someone is going to be reading or hearing what you wrote, the answers change. Of course, a trained professional is going to know how to sniff out these lies in a loving manner.

The point is: **the journal can only help if you are honest.** Because, after all, if you lie in the journal, you are just lying to yourself.

Next, don't stress about how much or how little information you write down. You don't have to carry a book around with you of all the calories, fats, proteins, and carbohydrates of every food known to man.

You can simply put an app (such as MyFitnessPal) on your smart phone and track your food intake. Or you can use a pen and paper and keep a log of what you eat, and *when.*

Be as accurate as you can when recording what you've eaten. Take a look at what you've eaten and see where you could have improved, and try to make better choices the next time you eat.

Remember that your goal is to make better choices, based on what you learn. Learning won't take forever. I know that doing anything *from now on* is hard to do.

If you tell someone they have to do something for a couple of weeks, it'll be pretty easy for them, but if you tell them they will have to do something for the rest of their lives, then it seems impossible.

Don't think keeping track of your food is something you will have to do forever. It may be good to do it again every so often, say, once a year or every six months, just to make sure you haven't slipped back into your old bad habits.

To start, I recommend keeping one for at least two weeks. If you are really motivated, and you do well with routine, then you could strive for one month. Since most of us have regular routines and patterns (whether we know it or not), you can find out a lot about yourself in two weeks.

When you are keeping your food journal, don't forget to include what you drink.

Track your coffee, tea, and sodas consumption (even the diet ones).

The average person takes in over 50000 calories a year from colas and other soft drinks. Here in the USA, keeping track of the amount is easy because they put the number of ounces right on the side of the cup.

Also, don't forget to record what you put into your coffee. The creamer, sweetener, or sugar *all count*. In many cases, we don't really think about things like this. Many people don't realize just how dangerous and detrimental their daily coffee fix is to their dieting success.

That's the point of a good journal. It's supposed to make you think.

The most important part of keeping a food journal *that works* is writing down what you were thinking and feeling at the time. For most of us, eating food isn't always a rational act.

We eat when we are tired, frustrated, angry, and bored. Some people even eat just because it gives them something to do with their hands. It's kind of like with smokers; they have to have busy hands!

You need to know *why* you are eating *what* you are eating.
This is another reason not to share your journal.

You have to feel free to write your emotions down, like how you felt when your boss gave you extra work to do right before you were going to leave for home. You have to feel free to vent about your husband, kids, dogs, etc. You also may not want everyone knowing you are routinely awake at three in the morning and eat because you are tired or because you are afraid to go back to sleep.

And just think about what your co-workers would think if they found out how you felt about them! You would make better food choices if they weren't always encouraging you to eat out or join them when they did.

By keeping a food and thought journal and analyzing it, you will eventually see patterns emerging.

You'll be able to tell what times during the day make you make your poorest food decisions. It may be that your second break after lunch, when you are feeling tired or sluggish, is your danger zone. Perhaps Friday afternoons are a problem because your small, planned reward for doing well throughout the week turns into a binge.
You can find out so much about yourself and why you are making the choices you do by keeping an honest journal.

It's Not the Cookie, It's the Bag

Diets don't work. They might work for a short while, but they will eventually cause you to return to your old, unhealthy eating habits and your old weight. In many cases, you will even gain a few more pounds.

The truth is this: just about any diet will give you short-term results, some better than others. The problem comes when you have to live with these choices. The body and, more importantly, the mind, rebels at being denied.

That is why I don't *diet*. For the most part, my weight loss efforts have consisted of sensible eating combined with regular exercise.

Of course, there are many myths about what passes as healthy eating.

Cutting out bad things like sodas, candy, potato chips, cookies, ice cream, etc. is not only discouraging, it's a recipe for disaster.

You already know that I had help with my weight loss as a result of having gastric surgery. This made a lot of my problems go away, but I still had to learn to make better food choices. During the years since this

25

procedure, I have learned one important thing about myself when it comes to those "bad foods."

I've learned that no one or very few of us can eliminate these items from their diet for good.

And I'm not sure it's a good idea to do even if you are one of those rare people who can pull it off. You would have to change so much that your personality would be totally different.

So, I've learned that I can't eat like I used to. But I also know that saying that I will never have another ice cream cone, candy bar, or bag of potato chips might affect my mood.

So how do you handle the dilemma of not depriving yourself verses overeating or even binging? The answer is in this book and chapter's title: IT'S NOT THE COOKIE, IT'S THE BAG!

Think about it for a minute.

How many cookies are there in a bag? How many of them could you eat without wrecking your health plans? Can you honestly say that you could have a whole bag of cookies in the house without eventually eating the whole bag?

My family's answer to this is where I got the idea for this book.

I live with my mom, my youngest brother, Patrick, his 17-year-old son, Seth, and our crazy dog, Penny. They have been a great help to me during this whole process. They plan the meals, do the shopping, read the confusing food labels, prepare the food, etc. But it's hard to tell a teenage kid that there won't be any cookies or ice cream in the house!

So, when making food decisions as a family, we compromised. Once or twice a week we buy a single package of frozen cookie dough. It makes just enough for us to each have four or five cookies. We satisfy our sweet tooth, but don't have the temptation of having three to six dozen cookies around. When we want ice cream, we get a half pint from the convenience store. It's more than one person should have, but we share it. When we make cornbread or French bread for a meal, we make only enough for that one dinner. If there happens to be leftovers, they go in the freezer. That means to have them you have to take them out, defrost them in the microwave, and then butter them for eating. This is a lot of work just to satisfy a craving!

Occasionally, they will bring home one candy bar and we will split it three ways. We sometimes do the same thing with a bag of miniatures.

When it's one of our birthdays, we still have a cake, but it's a smaller one that will be gone once everyone has had a slice.

When it comes to chips, we buy plain nachos to use with hummus, refried beans, or cheese. Trust me, it's harder to eat plain chips even with these helpers! But, again, we don't buy the huge bags. We buy the medium-sized ones. Then, even if one of us has a setback and eats more of them than they should; the bag is empty that much quicker.

During the holidays, we still make a pie. We don't have three or four or more of them; we have *one*. And whatever we don't eat is given away to friends or relatives as soon as possible.

Think about a box of Pop Tarts or a box of pudding cups. Again, you have many more than you need, and they are right there calling your name. Have you thought about buying one package of instant pudding mix, making it at home, and sharing it with your family? This is a better solution.

As you can see, the problem with most foods is the quantity in which they are sold or prepared.

Even for relatively healthy people, it's hard not to eat the whole bag of chips, finish off that carton of ice cream, or empty that bag of cookies. I know. Before I had the surgery I had even more trouble with these foods. Even now, cornbread and French bread are two of my weaknesses.

The real problem is that it's harder to have willpower when that great, tasty food you know you shouldn't want is right there in your pantry, cupboard, refrigerator, or freezer.

So, brainstorm about how you can solve this problem. What items do you enjoy eating that you could purchase or prepare in smaller quantities? Are there places you could buy just one cupcake or only four cookies?

Is there someone you know who would love to share a pie or batch of brownies the next time you make them so you won't have a whole pan staring you in the face or calling to you in your sleep? Is there a bakery that would sell you a half a loaf of French bread so you don't have to bake the whole loaf? Or could you freeze half of it and only bake what you really need?

Are there restaurants where you could go and buy one slice of pie or cake?

I ask these questions because I don't know where you live. I don't know what you have available to you. I live near a big city, and have a lot of options, but you may live in a small town with one store that isn't even open 24 hours.

The key point is to **reduce the quantity of treats you consume**. Because YOU WILL continue to consume them throughout your life. That's just a fact.

However, if you remember that it's not the cookie, it's the bag, you will have a greater chance of success in your weight loss journey.

Put Your Health on Your Schedule

In our busy, daily lives we all have many appointments and obligations. We make lists and follow schedules. We have planners and smart phone apps. We make a point to be on time, and to be prepared for events.

We use alarms and calendars to remind ourselves of special appointments like meetings with the boss, a doctor's visit, a hair appointment, or a special date night.

D0 you show as much care for your diet and exercise?

When you make out your daily calendar, do you pencil in time for exercise, prayer, or meditation? Is it important enough to carve out the time for it? Your exercise routine doesn't have to take a lot of time. My goal is 30 minutes, minimum, each day.

Could you find that small amount of time four to five days a week to improve your health? Is it important enough to you to actually put it on your calendar right along with all the *important things* in your life? Could you ever see yourself telling someone, "Sorry, I cannot make it to that appointment, because it's going to cut into my exercise time"? I haven't gotten to *that* point yet, but I do know that I feel worse when I don't have some form of daily activity.

I usually get my exercise by riding a stationary bike or by walking on a treadmill. While I am at it, I listen to audio books. I find this a great time to open my mind to the teachings of inspirational authors such as Wayne Dyer, Joel Osteen, Steven Covey, Norman Vincent Peale, Joyce Meyer, Jennifer Rothschild, and others.

How much thought do you put into what you will have to do, and eat, each day?

Do you plan any or all of your meals? Do you participate in the shopping? Have you spent any time educating yourself as to how to interpret the labels on food? Do you carry a lunch to work, or do you eat out? If you eat out, do you plan in advance where you will go and what you will have? Do you have any of the menus for your local restaurants, or are you familiar with what all they offer?

Between the stress of the work place and the responsibilities of home and family, most people just don't think about what they will have to eat each day. They grab whatever is handy, or they eat out of vending machines or coffee carts. I've been there myself. When I worked in the carnival, most things I ate were ones that could be eaten while still working in the crowds. Some of my favorites were hot dogs, corn dogs, popcorn, hamburgers, and Frito pies.

It wasn't until I quit traveling with the show that I finally started eating healthier. I'll admit that it's a lot easier when you don't have the pressure of time and deadlines. I work hard online, but I'm still working from home, so I have it a bit easier than most people do.

Have you thought about taking your lunch and snacks to work?

I know it's not easy to do this, because doing so often means getting up early or staying up a little later to prepare your meal. The bigger issue is what you should put in the lunch. There is a lot of advice on what is healthy and what isn't. Also, there is the issue of which is cheaper: making a lunch or eating out?

There aren't a lot of easy answers to these questions, but I do have some suggestions.

Nowadays, just about every restaurant has a website, a blog, or a Facebook or Instagram page. You can usually go there and find out what they offer for lunch. You can review the choices at your leisure and make as good of a decision as possible. You can also print these out and mark what you plan to order.

Because many of us have to eat fast food at some point in our week, the clinic where I had my surgery has all the major chain restaurant menus posted on their website, along with the calories and fat content and advice on which choices are your best bets.

Doing research ahead of time is great, because you can choose the best option out of the poor choices you have. Knowing in advance what you're going to order will help you to NOT make a rushed decision when at the counter or in the drive-thru lane.

Often it's not the concept of eating out that is the problem, it's not really caring about the choices you make. This comes from the erroneous belief that there is no good choice. There may not be a truly healthy alternative, but there are options that are better for you. You could choose to have a salad with your Big Mac instead of fries.

Another strategy to use is to share your desire to eat healthier with others. You can ask your co-workers or group to select a different restaurant that has better options for you. You may even learn that you aren't the only person who wants this! You may just be the only one who is willing to admit you are working to improve yourself.

If all else fails, you can certainly eat alone at a place that gives you a better chance to find a good selection. One other thing to remember about choosing what to have is that you don't have to be perfect. If you have a day where you really feel like having a greasy cheeseburger, this doesn't mean you are hopeless. It just means that tomorrow you will need to start over and try to do better.

Are you willing to keep certain items at work? There are a lot of things you can keep in your office or your car that will make staying on track so much easier. The first thing I would recommend is that you buy a water bottle and flavor mixers and keep them handy. Water is good for us, but most of us know it's not very tasty. When was the last time you said to yourself, *"Hey, I'm thirsty. I can't wait to get a tall glass of water!"*?

There are a lot of great low-calorie flavor mixers that you can use to make the taste of water enjoyable. Some of the top brands are Crystal Lite, Kool Aid, and Jolly Rancher. There are also many good store brands. I am a fan of Great Value products, sold by

Walmart and HEB. Their Orange Sunrise tastes like orange juice!

You may even get to the point that you favor water over a latte or a cappuccino. (I'm a coffee lover, so we both know *that* probably won't ever happen.) But every bottle or glass of water you drink puts you that much closer to your goal. It not only helps you avoid hunger, but it will help you improve your mood. And you won't be consuming the extra calories found in special coffee drinks.

Now let's talk about snacks.

High-protein, low-fat, low-carbohydrate snacks are best. Some of my favorites that can be consumed either at home or away from home are nuts, beef jerky, and dried fruit. Of course, you have to get freeze-dried fruit, as it has the lowest sugar content. Low-fat string cheese is excellent if you have access to a refrigerator.

While they aren't a perfect option, prepackaged cheeses or peanut butter with crackers aren't that bad. They are high in both protein and fat, so eating them might mean you'll get a few queer looks.

If you really want to make progress during your weight loss journey, then you have to be more worried about yourself than the thoughts of others. Trust me, there will be others who want to do what you are doing but just don't have the courage to put themselves first and do whatever it takes to lose the weight and keep it off.

Staying hydrated, eating better snacks, and taking charge of your meals are the kinds of things you will have to do to achieve the success you want for the long term.

Are you willing to take these few small steps? Is your health important enough to put it on your schedule? Are you willing to plan things out, like you would an important presentation? Are you willing to look a little silly to reach your goals?

These planned actions will all be worth it. I say this from experience. Since starting my path towards good health, I only started to make real progress in my business life once I committed myself to taking the daily actions required to get healthy and stay that way. Now, when I feel sluggish, I do some exercises. I am also trying to find a new way to be active. I am looking into yoga, Martial Arts, and ballroom dancing as examples of things I can learn to do. And instead of a candy bar or a fancy dessert, I seek out even healthier foods when I am feeling down.

Just wait until your colleagues see just how much more energy and passion you have once you decide to invest in yourself and get physically healthy!

6 Exercise Myths to Ignore

There are many reasons why people don't exercise. *But a lot of them are really just excuses!*

I'm going to talk about some of them and see if I can help you get past these blocks.

Myth #1: Exercise is hard!

People think that exercise has to be hard or take a long time. They think that if they aren't exercising for hours, they can't possibly see any results. And how many people refer to it as *working out*? We've all heard the old expression: *"No pain, no gain,"* right?

This may be a great mantra for a well-conditioned or generally healthy person wanting to push themselves and become even more toned, but for people who are seriously overweight, it's not a good way to think about your exercise time.

When you exercise, it should be as fun as you can possibly make it. Think about when you were a child. I'm sure you sometimes played for hours not realizing just how much energy you were burning. You didn't have to walk on a treadmill, ride a stationary bike, or use a rower.

Exercise that is painful is rarely repeated.

If you feel sore after exercising, then you probably did too much or perhaps you did the wrong kind of activity for your current physical condition. You may even have an underlying medical problem that you should address with your doctor.

For example, I am 50 years old, and starting to feel the pain of arthritis in my right shoulder, right knee, and lower back. My doctor advised me to take a Tylenol prior to exercising and to stagger my work-out so that it isn't as punishing to my body.

So, keep your exercise time as fun and pain-free whenever possible!

Myth #2: Exercise takes too much time!

Exercise takes time, but not as much time as you would think! It's all about doing something, taking action, and getting moving. Some of the most important steps are those few you take when you are just starting out. For some people, just the act of putting on their shoes and stepping outside their house is a victory.

It's those small, courageous first steps that will get you to your big goal. Anyone who runs marathons, participates in triathlons, or sets personal records in weight-lifting had to start with *one thing*. They had to start with one step, one lap, one mile, one sit-up, one bench press, one pull-up, one push-up, one *something*.

When you are just starting out, you won't be able to do *any* exercise no (matter how low-impact it is) for very long.

The first time I ever walked on a treadmill, I was scared to death. I had visions of the scene at the end of the Jetsons cartoons with me running for my life on a crazed piece of equipment. I walked at one mile per hour for five minutes and was worn out.

The next time I did it, I went for ten minutes. Eventually, I got to where I could do 15 to 30 minutes at a stretch at two miles per hour.

This reminds me of something that happened while I was making my regular trips to the clinic that did my surgery.

They are located in a building with two towers. When we first started going there, we would park in their garage so I wouldn't have to walk very far. Later, they would make changes to their garage, and there wouldn't be an easy place for us to park our big, four-door truck. What most people would do is park and then walk over from one building to the other using an overhead walkway.

In the beginning, I wasn't in good enough shape to make this walk. By the time I had to, I could do it, but only by stopping three or four times, because it's about a quarter of a mile in length.

Later, I would get to the point where I could not only walk it without stopping, but without being winded when we got there!

I'm now happy that I can make this walk, but the point I'm trying to make here is that *you don't have to work out for an hour or even 30 minutes to get the benefit of exercising.*

What you have to do is simply do as much as you possibly can… and then do *more* the next day. If you wait too long before exercising again, could injure yourself. You have to find a balance between challenging yourself and staying safe. So, what is *one* exercise you could start doing today? Can you do one push-up, one jumping jack, one curl, or one of something else? How about just putting on your shoes and stretching your muscles? Are there chores that you do most days or do every day that cause you to expend energy? Could you put on some music and dance?

Exercise doesn't have to be hard, boring, or take forever!

Besides, we all know the saying: "Time flies when you're having fun!"

It's true! So focus on having fun when you're moving your body!

Myth #3: You need proper work-out clothing in order to work out.

People always worry about how they look.

If you are seriously overweight, nothing looks good on you. Most work-out clothes look even worse, as many were designed to make good-looking, sexy people look even better. Some people think they have to have new clothes or shoes before they can really exercise properly.

Of course, *this isn't true*!

I've gotten a good sweat in blue jeans, sweat pants, shorts, and even pajamas. After all, most times I exercise, it's from the comfort of my own home. Remember, I'm blind, and I usually ride a stationary bike or walk on a treadmill.

Some people worry that they need new shoes. They claim they are afraid of hurting themselves if they don't have the proper footwear.

This is actually a very valid worry, because the truth is that wearing ill-fitting shoes can cause injury while working out. Shoes made specifically for a given activity are always best.

But here, again, we are talking about people who are in relatively good shape that are interested in going further. For someone in bad shape, you are not very likely to hurt yourself or do long-lasting damage because you don't have a new pair of Air Jordan's!

I often walk on my treadmill in shoes my mom wouldn't let me wear out of the house! It has never done me any harm. I walk somewhere between one and three miles per hour, depending on how I am feeling.

So, put on your ugliest, oldest, funkiest gear and just get moving! But get yourself a good pair of shoes that have support. This is necessary, and it will motivate you, too!

Now, I know you must be thinking that it's easy for me because I have a bike and a treadmill right in my home.

It is easier, true, but I need to mention a few points here, which leads me to my next exercise myth.

Myth #4: You have to have top-of-the-line equipment in order to work out.

First of all, let me say that there are people who have such equipment in their homes and still do not use it. I personally think one of the stupidest features on some exercise equipment is being able to fold it out of the way when not in use.

For those of you who have the gift of sight, it's better if you can see your equipment on a regular basis. Much better, in my opinion, because I imagine your equipment staring you in the face, guiltily asking: "Why you aren't using me?" If you can see it, you should use it!

There are also people who work at companies or live in buildings that have amazing exercise equipment but don't use it either. I know sometimes making it down to the basement or around to the clubhouse is a problem.

Another thing about my equipment is that *none of it is new*. It isn't even *close* to being new. I got both of them from my uncle, who is a marathon runner. (I think he secretly hopes that someday I'll join him in a 10-K race!)

He uses his equipment so hard, and he has a need for the latest models. So, when it's time to get new equipment, he gives me his old stuff, which is still useable!

Do you know *why* he gives it to me instead of one of his children or grandchildren? It's simple. **He knows I will use it.**

This leads to me to a great story I want to share with you.

When I was first starting on my road to better health, I didn't have *any* exercise equipment.

I was still traveling with my uncle's carnival, part-time. One night, we were at a Christmas Lights festival in Lake Jackson, Texas, and my nephew, Seth, went to a church rummage sale that was part of the festival.

I don't know if he bought it for me or for himself or just because it was something he could afford, but he bought an exercise bike for five bucks.

It was one of those old-style, torturer models with the small hard seat that very few people can ride without using a towel or a pillow on it. (I know you've seen them! Some of you have probably even used one!)

Well, Seth brought it home and set it outside our house on the sidewalk that runs between our house and the garage. I live near Houston, Texas, so we don't generally have harsh winters. However, where the bike was situated was where the wind would blow right at you.

I used that awful bike in that cold and wind. I rode it in the hot summer sun. I rode it during the day, and when the mosquitoes were biting at night.

I never missed a day.

There was an overhang, so rain didn't stop me. And, being blind, I couldn't see the distance or time I was using it. At first, I kept track of time by counting *one thousand and one, one thousand and two*, and so on. Later, I would use the sleep timer on my digital audio book player.

I believe it was my dedication to using this simple bike that made my uncle decide to give me his cast-off equipment.

I'm so glad he did! (Now, if he would just get a rower or stationary hand bike he doesn't need so I can start working on my upper body… that would be awesome!)

Do you know someone who has equipment they aren't using? Perhaps they can give it to you.

Maybe one of your relatives or friends received an elliptical, a recumbent bike, or a weight stack for a birthday or as a Christmas present and haven't used it. Maybe you could check Craigslist or one of the other free classified sites online to see what is out there.

I bet you know *someone* you could ask to make you their guest or their "plus one" on a health club membership. (Some companies provide such memberships for their employees.) Many insurance providers offer as much as "half off" on fitness center fees. You could check Goodwill or other charitable organizations that resell items. Most people like to help those who help themselves, so, if someone gives you work-out gear, the best way you can thank them is to use it!

Myth #5: You will always feel good about working out, and you will always be able to do so.

Regardless of how good you are doing with scheduling your exercise time, there will be times you don't, won't, or can't exercise as you would like.

I have had days where I didn't feel like getting out of bed... just like you've had at some point in your life. On those days you either decide to exercise later in the day or you give yourself a pass. You say to yourself, "I will do better tomorrow."

Now, you might also be thinking: "What if I start off on yet another exercise plan and fail to lose weight or keep it off?" I know quite often it's easier and more comfortable not to try than it is to risk failure. **The question you have to ask yourself is: "What am I more afraid of?"**

Are you more scared of failure... or of dying an early death and/or suffering with many illnesses and diseases caused by obesity?

Losing weight and keeping it off is a long, hard process. I had surgery, and it *still* took me almost four years to get to where I am at today.

And I fail all the time. But I prefer not to use that "f" word. I prefer to say that there are days when I am disappointed in myself or my progress. But I love myself enough not to beat myself up over it, and I know that every day is an opportunity to move just a little bit closer to where I want to be.

The same applies to you! Take one step at a time. If you fall, pick yourself up. It is really just that simple.

Myth #6: You will be laughed at by everyone.

Nothing could be further from the truth. Yet big people are afraid others will laugh at them. It's a fact of life that often the skinny, seemingly-perfect people will make fun of someone who is severely overweight. Then there is the perception that no one would be that fat if they didn't want to be. You are accused of being lazy or weak. Sometimes, this is obvious, and other times, it's just the feeling you get.

So, you have to decide for yourself what is most important to you. Are you more worried about how you will look or how you will feel? Are you willing to be laughed at or stared at in order to get healthy?

Are you willing to put in hard work, and then look back at your old self and say, "Heck, yeah, I was a mess, but I did something about it!"?

Remember, just four years ago, I was a mess, too.

I weighed 512 pounds on February 14th, 2012. And my brother has an earlier photo of me where he swears I look to be about 600 pounds. I was on seven prescription medicines, taking twelve pills a day. I had high blood pressure and was borderline Diabetic. But I made the decision to change.

No one laughed at me. Instead, they encouraged me and helped me and they still do.

Now, I am admired for what I have accomplished, and you will be admired, too!

Now that I have eliminated all your exercise excuses and debunked the most popular exercise myths, I hope you will be getting out there and taking action.

I hope you realize that it's more about what you do—*no matter how little it may seem to you at the time*—that really and truly matters. **Anything you do will be a step forward, and will bring you closer to your goal of good health.**

I really want you to succeed. People tell me all the time that I take away their excuses. I've heard, *"If the blind guy can do it, then why can't I?"* on more than one occasion! They tell me I inspire and motivate them to do more and be a better person. I hope that I can do this for you when it comes to your exercise. I want to help you write a new chapter of your life... a story of strength, courage, power, and good health.

Now get moving, and take your first step!

Strengthen Your Support System

It's widely known that we can accomplish much more with the help of a team than we can on our own.

I firmly believe that the reason people are successful is because they have a solid team behind them. It may be made up of friends, family members, coworkers, employees, or people with similar interests or problems.

Nowhere is this truer than with issues of health. I'm specifically talking about weight loss here, but it also applies to people suffering from addictions like alcohol and drugs—both prescription and illegal.

We need the help of others to keep ourselves motivated and inspired. We also need them to provide additional information, advice, and suggestions.

The people who are going to help and support you are those who will make up your support system.

When it comes to healthy eating, effective exercise, and using vitamin supplements, there is so much to learn and absorb. There are so many sources for information that you have to decide which among them work and which are just another attempt to use your need to lose weight to separate you from your money.

My best advice to you is to begin strengthening your support system by seeing just who you have in your existing circle that can help you succeed.

Talk to your friends, your family, your health care providers, your co-workers, and your online friends (provided you are online, on social media, in some form or another!).

Reach out to anyone who will help and support you in your weight loss journey. You'll be surprised at how receptive and wonderful people can be when they learn of your plan to successfully lose weight and keep it off!

I know one of the things that really impressed me with the TLC (Texas Laparoscopic Consultants) is that they are invested in the lives of their patients. One thing my surgeon, Dr. Scarborough, told me at our first meeting was this: "Once you are one of our patients, you are a patient for life. You become part of our extended family." This applies to everyone that comes to see them, even the ones who aren't good candidates for a gastric procedure. And I believe they sincerely mean this when they say it. As a result, they require you to attend diet and nutrition classes prior to the surgery. They also insist that you speak with a psychologist to make sure you are emotionally ready to make the lifestyle changes required to be successful.

After the procedure, you are scheduled for regular checkups. They start on a monthly basis and are only extended after they are convinced you are making the expected progress. Then the visits will stretch to every other month, then every three months, and then every six months.

They monitor all kinds of information on you through regular bloodwork. I routinely have ten or more vials of blood taken from me prior to each appointment. And they were the ones who noticed that my white blood count was elevated and insisted I see a hematologist. This led to many more tests, including a colonoscopy.

The result was that I was diagnosed with a disease called CLL, Chronic Lymphocytic Leukemia. As my oncologist says, it sounds worse than it is. It basically means that my white blood cells don't die off like they are supposed to. Instead, they build up in the body. CLL is something that you can live a long time with and never know you have it. It is still in the very early stages, and my doctors tell me to expect to live a long, healthy, fruitful life. That's what I am planning on doing.

Do you have a doctor that you trust to share all your worries with? Can you tell him or her about your struggles with weight? Have you ever asked if they could help you by referring you to a dietician, nutritionist, or therapist? Your doctor can be a valuable asset, but you have to trust them enough to communicate with them openly and honestly. You also have to be committed to doing whatever it takes to finally lose the weight and keep it off.

Another thing that impressed me about the clinic was their dedication to support groups. They have monthly meetings of clients. There are both online and in-person groups. In each, you share stories, recipes, successes, and disappointments. They also have an email list and a Facebook group. They encourage you to lean on your family and friends for support and encouragement.

There are such groups for just about any interest or problem. I'm sure you have heard of weight loss groups on Facebook or Google Plus. You may even belong to one or more of them.

Are they the kinds of places that encourage your progress? Do you openly discuss problems you are having? Have you ever been truly helped by one of their members?

A group can only help you if you use it. If you aren't interacting on an honest, authentic basis, then you can't expect to get the answers you need. And you certainly can't get the inspiration and motivation that you need if you don't use it!

If you are on social media, one thing to consider when you start a new diet or fitness plan is whether or not you are going to share it online.

Should you post photos or report on your progress? For many people, this is scary. The fear of failure might hold you back. The fear of others being disappointed with you might prevent you from wanting to be openly public about what you're doing. You might feel afraid that others will laugh or post mean things about you. This is a possibility, but so many people struggle with the problem of weight loss or with some other equally troublesome issue that most people will be generous and sympathetic towards you—as long as you write your posts with an attitude of humility and thankfulness. Be sure people know you aren't bragging.

Another thing you should know is that most people want to see you succeed. Heck, they want to see *anyone* they know succeed!

I am still surprised that my most active posts on social media are about my health. At Christmas time, I posted a photo of me and my dog by my Christmas tree. I got many great comments on that one, and it made me feel so good inside! It also reminded me that I have to keep it up. Knowing that people are watching can be a good thing. I didn't lose the weight for anyone but me, because I knew it was a matter of getting healthy or I'd die.

But I'm not saying you would or should lose the weight you need to because of what other people will think. The simple truth is knowing that you have an audience who is watching you and cheering you on, can be a great motivator. It can give you the strength to get out of bed early to do some extra exercise. It can motivate you to choose yogurt instead of ice cream or water instead of a foamy latte.

The point having a group to cheer you on when you do well and console you when you fall short is a big factor in your success or failure at getting healthy and staying that way. So, I urge you to share on Facebook, or on other social media.

Post your starting weight along with your goal and a request for help along the way. Tell your friends online and off that you know it will be hard and you will be depending upon them to help keep you going.

Then post regular updates, sharing your successes and setbacks. Tell them where you think you went wrong and ask for suggestions. Announce what steps you are taking to remedy the problem that caused you to backslide.

Post the occasional photo. They don't have to be swimsuit photos (and probably won't be!) but they should be good photos. I find that my friends could tell I was making progress even when I wore my regular jeans and pullover. You can even post *before* and *current* photos, once you are on your way.

When I posted my *before* and *after* photos for anniversaries or milestones, my friends were amazed with my progress. I had over 200 pounds to lose.

Whether you need to lose that "extra ten pounds" or you are morbidly obese, the truth is *you can only lose the weight and keep it off with the help of others (and some dedication!).*

If you don't have anyone who will support you in your efforts, then seek me out. I am on Facebook, LinkedIn, Google Plus, and Twitter. My social media and contact information are all in the *About the Author and His Books* section of this book.

So, how strong is your support network? If you have a good one in place, then why aren't you using it? Or are you?

If you don't have anyone that will support you, then get out there and join some support groups, whether they are in person or online.

If you are already a member of such a group, then start showing up and letting them help you make progress towards becoming the healthy person you want to be.

I couldn't have done it by myself. I also wouldn't be able to maintain my weight by myself, without all of the support I have received and still receive.

I openly admit this… and I'm proud to admit it.

I have to thank my doctors, their staff, my family, those friends online who are almost like family, my social media networks, and people who I don't even know who have all said, "Max, you can do it!" or "Max, you are doing great!" or, best yet, "Max, you look awesome!"

By strengthening your support system, you will be more likely to achieve the results you want and feel good about yourself.

Use Modern Meditation

Do you meditate?

Have you considered adding this practice to your daily routine? Have you ever tried to meditate but found it difficult to add it to your daily routine, and make it a regular practice?

I ask because there are definite health benefits to using meditation.

Personally, I believe it works, and have used it myself. **However, I have a broader definition of what meditation is and how it can be practiced.**

When you think of meditation, you probably think of a ritualized process with a lot of rules. You might have read internet articles or books to find out the proper means of meditation and the ideal length of time a person should meditate to receive the health benefits.

To me, the whole point of meditation is to focus. The idea is to find something to center your mind on so that you can block out everything else.

I also believe that listening to your body and focusing on your breathing are key parts of successful meditation. You don't have to have be in a specific room or chant meaningless words to focus your mind and spirit. The idea of picturing yourself in a calm place might not work for you, but that is okay.

The thing about meditation is that you can find a lot of opportunities and locations for your thoughtful reflection and concentration practices, and incorporate them into your day.

Here are some examples from my own life.

I have a dog named Penny. She believes that when she is itchy or in need of some petting, I must drop everything I'm doing and scratch her. I used to get angry when that would happen. She often interrupted me while I was in the middle of something. There aren't a lot of things I do well with just one hand. I couldn't write a blog post, reply to my emails, and post on social media, etc., while I was petting her.

I finally decided to take advantage of these interruptions, and I now look forward to her breaking into my day.

For anywhere from five to thirty minutes, I scratch her back, rub her belly, and stroke her fur. I focus on the repetitive motions and the warmth of her body.

I think about the pleasure I am bringing her. I slow my thoughts and focus on my breathing. I get a sense of calmness and I relax for a short time.

If you have pets, then stop thinking of attending to them as chores and start seeing this as an opportunity to close off your mind and slow yourself down.

This could apply whether you are scratching a dog, stroking a cat, grooming a horse, etc.

There are many times in our day we could use to improve our mental health if we just allow ourselves to enjoy the moment.

For example, when you take a bath or shower, are you just trying to get clean or do you take some time to relax your mind and body? I personally think that one of the reasons why women have less stress and live longer than men is because it's socially acceptable for them to enjoy a long, hot bath—with scented bath salts, candles, music, and even wine.

In 2014, I went to a conference where I had access to a tub. Because I had been so overweight for so long, it had been *forever* since I soaked in a tub. I gratefully sank down into it, letting my body settle and feel the warmth seep into my body. I focused on the steam and breathed deeply. I took much longer than I should have... and actually wished I had had someone who could scrub my back!

At home, I use a shower. When I go in there, I stay until the hot water runs out. I let the spray beat down on my head, neck, shoulders, and back. I breathe in the steam and listen to the water pound against my body or the walls of the shower. Yes, I am blessed with a great bathroom and just enough hot water. But I also sing in the shower. I sing loud and with passion. I sing songs my voice isn't capable of outside the shower. I can reach notes well out of my range more in the bathroom than in any other room.

When I dry off, I use a fresh towel, and I drink in the scent of the fabric softener and detergent used in the laundry. If I shower before bedtime, nothing is better than wallowing in the smell of freshly laundered sheets as you put your head on the pillow.

You can see that I have taken a relatively ordinary thing most people do every day

and made it special. My bathroom has become a place to block out all the noise and grab at least fifteen minutes of silence and find peace in myself.

Another time you can find this focus and peace is while doing a mindless, repetitive job or task or while exercising!

Think about the things you do in your daily life. Do you work at a job that requires you to perform the same tasks over and over again (such as at a factory or in an assembly line)? Do you spend time doing repetitive exercises?

That time you spend walking on the treadmill, climbing on a stair-master, paddling on a rower, pushing your upper body on a hand bike, or using an elliptical machine *could all* be opportunities for what I call modern meditation.

How long do you usually spend doing your exercise? While doing it, what are you focused on? Are you grumbling about having to exercise? Or are you getting in tune with your body? How do you feel when you find that perfect speed and rhythm that lets you feel like you, your body, and the machine are in harmony? Do you ever get to a point where you block everything out and just focus on your movements and your breathing?

Next time you are at the gym, try focusing on your breathing and concentration, and see if it makes your work-out go much easier.

Use your breathing to center yourself, and block out all the other noise around you. Don't think about the other patrons, the noise of the other machines, the work you aren't getting done because you are exercising, or the fun things you could be doing instead.

Just think about how much better you will feel for having exercised! Focus all your thoughts on breathing in and breathing out until you are the only person there.

The same thing can happen while doing menial work on an assembly line. I'm told that a lot of that equipment has a rhythm to it. You can use the labor to center yourself.

Once you get in the habit of doing what I call modern meditation, you could later move on to a more formal approach to it. I learned a lot about meditation from my dad, although I didn't realize that this was what he was doing at the time. My dad was one of those people who never let stress affect him.

He had several of his own methods.

One, he played the guitar. Often, I would hear him playing chords, running up and down the scales, or just playing favorite riffs over and over again. I now realize that he was doing these exercises more to think than to become a better musician.

Two, he liked to drive. You would think it strange for a man who drove thousands of miles a year to want to clear his mind by getting in the truck and going on a drive for pleasure, but that's what he did.

I now understand that he was using the scenery and the hum of the engine to focus his mind. I also figured out that the reason he used to ask me to go along with him was to have someone who could maybe help change a tire if needed but who wouldn't need to fill the cab with a lot of useless chatter.

Third, my dad would spend time around bodies of water. His favorite was the ocean. I recently learned that scientists deem there to be health benefits by being around the ionized air that you encounter near pounding surf. However, my dad could also feel at peace by being near a slowly moving river or a North Carolina mountain creek.

Our most important lessons are usually learned from watching or being around people we love rather than anything they tell us directly. I can thank my dad for teaching me about dealing with stress. He wouldn't have called it meditation, but that's what it was!

I now wonder if we would do more things that are good for us if we didn't always have to have names for them. Or maybe we should just choose less intimidating names! Some people dislike the word "exercise," and associate it with a negative chore. Perhaps calling it your "improvement time" or "meditation time" might be something to consider!

My goal is to help you get healthy.

I'm less interested in style or form and more interested in you reaping the benefits of meditation, *wherever, wherever,* and *however* possible!

There are definite health benefits to regular meditation.

Meditation allows you to reduce stress, lower blood pressure, increase focus, improve your mood, and encourage you to make better choices.

The problem isn't whether or not meditation works; the problem is how to implement it in a fast-paced, multi-tasking, never-enough-time world.

By using some of the simple yet unique strategies outlined in this chapter, you will begin to start reaping the rewards meditation provides.

Make Peace with Your Mirror

In 2015, I was interviewed for an article in New York Magazine. The writer asked an interesting question. She wanted to know how a blind person could appreciate the results of losing over 250 pounds.

I love questions that show the person asking them has tried to put themselves in your shoes. She imagined—correctly—that I can't look in a mirror. I also can't look at past photos of myself and compare them to ones of me today.

My scale will tell me my weight, but without some reference point, that number is just a number. I know my clothes are smaller now, but we threw out all my old clothes, so I can't even hold an old pair of jeans up to my waist to feel them to understand my progress.

I have had to depend on friends and family to tell me just how great I look and how well I am doing. As I mentioned in the last chapter, I like to post *before* and *after* photos on Facebook and other social media sites on key anniversaries for me just to have people tell me how much weight I have lost and how great I am doing. My favorite is when people, especially women, tell me I look hot! (Wink, wink!)

As to her question, I told her that I am no longer afraid of ramps or stairs. When I was at my heaviest, I avoided ramps altogether and went up and down steps like an old man.

When I go to the doctor, I can now get up and down from the table much easier. This is great because the doctor and her staff were always worried I would fall and hurt myself.

I avoided going places where I would have to walk a long distance. Now, if my family needs to park a long way from the entrance to a store or a doctor's office, I can easily walk there without losing my breath.

I can now buckle my seat belt with ease. Before, I either had to have an extension or just drape it over my arm hoping the police wouldn't see it. I've gone from wearing size 62 jeans and 4 XL tall shirts to fitting into size 40 pants and 2 XL tall shirts.

These are some of the ways I know I have changed without being able to look into a mirror.

This got me to thinking about how sighted people view their bodies and if there is something I could suggest that would help them with their progress.

It all comes down to how you see yourself when you look in the mirror.

I know this isn't a brand new idea, but maybe a blind guy can bring some new approach to it that will help you move forward.

The first place to start is to answer this question: Are you healthy?

I don't mean: *Are you perfect?*

I don't even mean: *Are you at the "ideal weight" for your height, age, and body type?*

What I mean is: *Are you healthy enough to participate in the activities you love or have always loved?*

Are you in good enough shape to play golf or tennis, chase the kids or grandkids, or walk the malls on Black Friday? If you are, then that is great! It doesn't mean you couldn't be in even better shape if you wanted to be.

There are quite a lot of people out there who are in pretty good shape who are trying to lose weight. They are doing it because they believe they should be skinnier.

They have looked at the tabloids in the checkout line at the grocery store and have seen the amazing women and men pictured on the front covers of magazines.

They have seen their favorite stars on the big screen nude or semi-nude and marveled at their perfection.

They have watched music videos and seen the teenaged stars mostly young girls in their skimpy attire strutting on screen.

They may have even heard from an unfeeling spouse that their sex lives would be better if the other partner made an effort to improve their looks.

These examples don't take into consideration the images and thoughts running through your mind when you stand in front of your mirror. This is why I started by asking if you were physically healthy.

If you know you are in good health, then it makes it far easier to resist all the voices that are constantly telling you aren't good enough, pretty enough, or sexy enough... and never will be.

I'm tempted to tell you to just avoid mirrors, but we all know that isn't practical. Even if you didn't have to use them when brushing your teeth, combing your hair, putting on makeup, trying on clothes, or shaving, it wouldn't be healthy.

So... you need to make peace with your mirror!

You have to be able to look into one and see the best *you* possible.

This isn't easy. You have to constantly tell yourself that you are a beautiful, sexy person.

Do this daily! It's easier to find things we are looking for, and if we look into a mirror expecting to see a god or goddess, then we are more likely to find our reflection pleasing to the eye.

If we cringe before looking because we just know a hideous monster will appear there, then we are far more likely to see the negative parts of our body.

No one is perfect. Everyone has flaws. Some people ignore theirs, and others choose to focus on their good traits.

Like the scale, the mirror is just a tool. It's not inherently good or bad. It won't lie to you. However, it will reflect what you see in your heart and mind.

If you still fear your mirror, you may want to temporarily cover it. Or you may want to remind yourself to not look at it before or after certain times of the day.

Since everyone looks better in lower light, you could consider changing the bulbs or fixtures in your bathroom (or whichever room that contains your mirror). Or you could mimic the visually impaired and wear a blindfold.

Spending some time without looking at your reflection may be just what it takes to accept that you are beautiful.

There are a lot of people who are overweight who still look good. Most of these people are that way because they have a confidence in themselves that others do not. They also carry themselves differently and usually dress with their best and worst features in mind.

So, stand up straight and hold your head up high. Stick your chest out and say, *"Hey, world, I'm a wonderful special person."* **Then decide to do the work every day to look and feel even better.**

I'm not perfect. My hair is greying and I have a small bald spot on the top of my head.

When my mom or brother point it out, I say, "Hey, no one would notice if you didn't mention it!"

After all, I am 6 feet, 4 inches tall. As long as I stay away from basketball games, who is going to notice? And my dad once told me that Ivey men either "go grey or go bald, so be thankful for the grey."

I am thankful for it. I have thick, naturally curly hair and have no desire to color it. I am truly happy with it.

However, I'm at the top end of normal on the BMI (body mass index) scale. I have fat left on me on my stomach, back, but, legs, arms, and shoulders. I am currently seeking some new exercises that will help me reshape what is left.

I could be unhappy with all of this, but I'm not. I'm in the best shape of my life!

Even going back to when I was a teenager, I've never been this healthy. I was well over 300 pounds in high school.

There is nothing that says you can't want to improve a body you are happy with. Just because someone owns a beautiful Corvette doesn't mean they can't want to add more chrome, change the paint, replace the tires, or upgrade the stereo and speakers.

If you know you are special, then the mirror can't tell you any different. If you believe you are pretty, then no one can convince you that you aren't.

If you think you or some part of you is ugly, then no one can make you feel better about it. I get up every day knowing I am very special but committed to maintaining what I have and improving upon it.

I would love to be able to look in a mirror. I can't. I can only listen to what people say. It's really good that I know my worth and will never let anyone tell me any different. I hope you can get to the point where you are as sure of yourself in this area!

I hope this has helped you to become more accepting of your body and be on better terms with your mirror. **You can make peace with your mirror by using positive affirmations (which were briefly touched upon in this chapter but will be discussed in-depth in the following one).** By repeating positive affirmations each day, you will unleash their full power and be able to change your views regarding your self-image in ways you never thought possible!

Use Positive Affirmations

You have probably heard about using affirmations to help you change your outlook and improve your life. If you haven't, I will teach you what to do. It is well-documented that they truly work. There is both religious and medical proof that positive affirmations are effective for people who can commit to using them.

Affirmations are positive statements that are repeated on a daily basis that alter your current (usually negative) beliefs by sinking into your subconscious.

While they initially may not be true, the constant repetition of them eventually makes them a reality—or so the theory goes.

However, I think others make it sound way too easy. I mean, it's one thing to go around thinking, believing, and speaking positive energy over your life when you are a success or when your life is going well, but what do you do when everything around you and everything you have ever been taught says you are a worthless failure and you should just be happy with what you do have?

I'm going to give you an approach to using affirmations that will really work.

This approach came to me when thinking about a time from my childhood. I was living in South Carolina and going to a new school because my dad had moved us there to be closer to the "Ivey" side of the family. There was an old-fashioned see-saw (teeter-totter) in the playground area. I would sit on it, but could never go up and down because, quite frankly, I was just too fat.

One day, some of the kids wanted to see how many of them it would take to raise me up. I don't know how many kids it took, but every inch of the opposite bar was covered. It was fun for just a second, feeling the thrill of going up and down. Then they laughed at me. I realized it was a big joke, and I cried about it.

I don't tell you this story to get your sympathy. One, because I'm no longer that person. I'm a physically healthy guy in the best shape of his life. I love my body, and others tell me I can be proud of it and the work that it took to get here. Two, because I want you to see that if you add enough goodness to one side it will balance out the bad on the other.

Maybe you aren't ready to go around saying "I am amazing, I am talented, I get whatever I go after, I have all the money I need," etc.

Maybe you grew up with parents who constantly told you were ugly, fat, stupid, clumsy, or a mistake. Maybe nothing you have ever tried has been a success. Maybe no one has ever come along to tell you just how special you are. The answer now is to start with what you **can** do.

First, when you have a negative thought, try not to speak it out loud. I know that our thoughts are with us all day long. The things we say to ourselves in our heads are often much worse than anything anyone else will say to our faces. But voicing these thoughts out loud gives them power. It makes the hurt far more painful and more difficult to overcome.

Try to catch yourself before blurting these hurtful thoughts out loud. Whenever you stop yourself from thinking or saying something hurtful, you make the job of balancing your life and your emotions so much easier. But if you can't stop yourself, then the next best thing to do is to balance them out with positive thoughts, words, and energy.

From now on, follow every negative statement up with at least *one* positive statement. If you burn the toast, and you yell *I am so stupid,* follow it up with *I am intelligent but am trying to do too many* *things at once*. If you look in the mirror, and say *I am so ugly*, then balance that out by saying *I am beautiful*.

Tell yourself: *I have many quality traits. I have great beauty. It just hasn't been seen by people who can appreciate my beauty.*

If you start the day by asking yourself: *Why am I always so tired?* Tell yourself: *I am an energetic person. I have all the energy I need to accomplish all of my tasks with joy and ease.*

Eventually, you *will* get to the point where you follow a negative with a whole string of positive thoughts and words.

I want you to get to the point where you eliminate the negative thoughts and words from your life altogether. I want you to see yourself as a wonderful, blessed, amazing human being.

Believe that you are the person you want to be. You know that there is a version of yourself that you were *meant* to become. And you know some or most of the things you need to do to become that person.

Learning how to remove the negative self-talk from your life and replacing it with positive, uplifting, empowering affirmations is a huge step towards becoming your ideal self.

Because your goal here is to lose weight and keep it off, this change in your outlook through positive thoughts and words will be a powerful tool in your journey to become healthier and get to your best weight.

The best affirmations are those that you create yourself.

If they are created through your own words and come from your own life experience, then you are more likely to repeat them to yourself and say them out loud.

Since their real power comes from constant repetition, it is important to use words and phrases that you can see yourself saying over and over again.

Here are a few good examples of affirmations for better health that you can use:

I *am* becoming the beautiful, healthy person that I am meant to be.

I *will* find the time and energy to exercise at least 15 minutes every day.

I *can* learn what foods are best for my body and reaching my ideal weight.

I *won't* let the people in my life keep me from eating healthier.

Tonight, I *will* get seven hours of restful, energizing sleep that will give me the energy I will need tomorrow to attack my goals.

I *have* the strength to do one more thing, and I am going to do it now.

I *am* going to eat healthy foods today.

I *am* a beautiful, sexy, desirable person.

Over time, you *will* start to believe these affirmations, even if you initially do not.

Now that we have talked about ending negative self-talk and replacing it with positive, loving affirmations, we need to address the other voices in your world.

Who do you surround yourself with? Do you hang out with positive people who are taking action in their lives and responsibility for their happiness? Or are your friends mostly negative, depressed, *going nowhere* types of people? The old saying is true: if you lie down with dogs you will wake up with fleas.

The people you surround yourself with can either support and encourage you or drag you down with them.

As your confidence in yourself grows, you will probably start to feel conflicts with many of the people you have known for a long time and with whom you routinely associate. You will have to decide which is more important: your good health and spiritual progress, or the comfort of an old friend who does not have your best interests at heart. I know it isn't easy to stop hanging out with people you have known for years. But you can start by inviting some new friends who are healthy into your life. This will balance your life out. The best case scenario would be to remove the negative, toxic people from your life altogether, but if you aren't ready to do that, then an alternative is to speak to them and make it known that you aren't going to allow them to speak hurtful noise in your presence.

Don't allow them to say mean, defeatist things to you, about you, or about themselves in your presence. This isn't being mean to *them*; it's being loving to *yourself*.

You can only allow so much negative energy into your life before it starts to affect you and keep you from your goals. Ideally, we would have no one in our lives that isn't supportive of us and our goals and dreams, yet I know this isn't practical. However, you can limit it as much as possible and you can balance it out with as many positive people and as much powerful energy as possible.

We can't keep out all the darkness and rain, but we can sure keep ourselves happier by letting in as much sunshine as we can find!

For example, I have a brother who I live with. He is very passionate about sports and politics. Sometimes, I have to put on my headphones, close the door to my room, or go out to the garage to get some time away from him. He isn't always the most positive person. Yet, I find that the more time he spends around me, the better he has become. He knows I'm a very positive person and that I won't stand for anyone putting themselves down in my presence. He knows that I will point out the good in a bad situation. I have more practice at it than he does, but he's learning.

Your friends and family will either learn or they will stop coming around you as much.

To be successful at *anything*, you have to have a lot of help. You need all the positive voices in your head you can get. You need people who will encourage and support you or help you solve your problems.

You don't need people saying, "You've failed over and over again so why are you even trying to lose weight now?"

I encourage you to invite at least one new, uplifting person into your life—even if you have to ask someone you know online.

I find the blogosphere very supportive and helpful, so maybe it's a great place for you to find such a friend.

I hope you will continue to do things like this to balance your life and give you a chance for real long lasting success.

Sometimes, we are so stuck in our own image of ourselves that we can't find the positive. Sometimes, it takes the clear vision of a loving friend to show us just how special we are and help us start the process of improving our self-image and changing our self-talk.

I know you think that I am a very self-assured person, but there are areas where I lack confidence in myself. For example, it took months before I would believe my friends who were telling me to share my story more.

They kept telling me that my life was very inspirational. I didn't see myself as anything special. I simply thought I was a guy who shows up every day and works his butt off to build a business that will allow him to support his family. I thought I didn't do anything special—I just find a way to accomplish the next task in front of me, whatever that may be.

I have learned how to do a lot of things I had never tried before *simply because I had to*. I didn't have anyone to do them for me and couldn't afford to hire someone either. My friends finally convinced me that I am special. They explained that there are so many people out there who have no physical disability who fail to take action to improve their lives or live the ones they do have.

I now realize just how big a deal it is to be one of the few that goes after his goals even when they are hard... but I wouldn't have seen this in myself without some great friends!

I started taking steps to share my story and help inspire others. I wrote and self-published my first e-book, *Leading You Out of the Darkness into the Light: A Blind Man's Inspirational Guide to Success*. I've written guest posts and been interviewed for a major magazine. I've done podcasts, radio shows, and online summits. I am not sharing this to brag, but to show what can happen when you change how you see yourself. Once you start to get a different picture of who you are *and just how special you really are*, you will start to think better thoughts, use better words, and take more positive action.

You will not only do more and think better of yourself, but you will find new parts to your personality. You will discover new talents, abilities, and skills. You will find you have the ability to learn many new things. And you will see more opportunities open up. This will happen partly because you are open to them, but mainly because everyone who comes in contact with you will be able to sense that you are a *living, growing, adapting, expanding, achieving* kind of person.

I hope this brings home the value of having great friends around you. I haven't changed. I'm still the same person I was before. The difference is that now I appreciate just how special I am. This is something that happened because I had people in my life (online and off) who wanted good things for me. They saw the best in my personality and convinced me of it. I would still be working hard without their encouragement because that is who I am, but I wouldn't have realized just how special I am without their help.

No matter how good a team is, they still need cheerleaders and coaches to remind them of their abilities and urge them to do even better in the future.

Who do you have in your circle of friends? Are they cheering you on?

Are they helping you move forward or dragging you backwards?

I hope you will follow my example here and not only bring some great new people into your life but listen to them when they tell you just how amazing you are.

By using positive affirmations, and repeating them each day, you will change your outlook and gain the confidence you need in order to move forward and achieve your goals.

Don't Be Afraid of Your Scale!

Are you afraid of your scale?

Do you dread stepping onto it?

Is weighing yourself the thing you hate most about visiting your doctor? Do you weigh yourself in the nude or deduct the estimated weight of your clothes from the number the scale says?

Do you weigh after you exercise or exit a sauna hoping the number will be lower? Have you even used the bathroom prior to weighing yourself, thinking that would make you lighter?

We do all kinds of crazy things when it comes to our weight.

How would you feel if your weight were broadcasted to everyone in the room?

Well, that is an experience that I have to live with. As a blind person, I can't avoid it. I either have to have someone tell me my weight, or I have to use a talking scale.

When I go to the doctor, everyone can hear my blood pressure, pulse, temperature, and weight. At home we have a talking scale, but there isn't room for it in our bathroom. It ended up in our dining room at the edge of the living room and kitchen. This means everyone in the house knows what everyone else weighs.

This can be good or bad.

Some people do well knowing that they have people watching. This is why groups like Weight Watchers have some success for a lot of people.

Others suffer from anxiety when they know anyone other than themselves will hear their weight. Some will even take extreme measures to ensure that their weight will go down before the next group meeting. I think knowing that my weight is not a secret—and never will be—has gone a long way to making me more comfortable with stepping on my scale in the first place.

That's where you want to get to.

You want to use the scale as the tool it was intended to be. It has only one purpose, to tell you your weight at a given time on a given day.

Your scale is not evil, and it isn't staring at you with distain when you add an ounce or a pound or two. It won't cheer your name or tell you how good you did when you lose weight, either. It is an inanimate object. It doesn't have the ability to call your friends or go on the internet and tell everyone when you had a setback (although some well-meaning computer programmer may change this at some point in the future!).

How often do you—or should you—weigh yourself? The experts say we should only weigh ourselves once a week on the same day at the same time. Of course, very few people are capable of keeping such a routine. We have been so conditioned to want and expect immediate results that it's hard to go a whole week without checking your progress.

I realize that it's far easier to go days without checking when you are in a good weight range. I often go several days at a time without getting on a scale. You know why the experts advise against weighing daily? It's because your weight will fluctuate, usually within 3 to 7 pounds! Even if you stick to a strict diet and exercise regimen, your weight will go up and down. I have had weeks where I exercised more than usual only to weigh myself and find my number went up.

There are a lot of things that can impact how our body processes the food we take in.

Even the amount of sunlight you get or don't get can have an impact on you.

By only weighing yourself once a week, you are less likely to be fooled into thinking you are doing really good or really bad. If you are committed to getting on that scale every morning, then you need to accept that the number isn't scientific. You need to accept whatever the number is and decide to be okay with it. You need to think of it kind of like how some people read their horoscope. It may or may not be true.

Regardless, you shouldn't let what your scale says ruin your life. In baseball there is an old saying about bad calls: *It will all come out in the wash.* What this means is that over a long season that lasts 162 games, the number of bad calls against you and good ones for you will balance out. Because of this old saying, ball players and managers don't get as upset as often at the bad calls when they come. Sure, if it happened in the heat of the moment in a critical game there might still be a brawl, but, for the most part, their outlook is: *We'll get 'em next time!*

This is the approach you have to take with weighing and how you use your scale.

Do not be afraid of your scale!

Once you weigh yourself, does the number on your scale effect how you think and act for the rest of the day?

Are you more attentive to your family or friendlier to your coworkers when your weight does down? Is your temper shorter when it goes up? Do you notice more things wrong with yourself, your home, your car, or your family when you have gained weight?

Most of us do. Our weight is a big part of our self-worth. We have been convinced that if our weight isn't where we believe it should be, such as at the ideal for our height, age, and body type, that we are somehow a failure. The truth is that you have to come to terms with what is a healthy weight for *you*. This can be determined with the help of a medical doctor or by using the body mass index (BMI) scale.

However, even this tool isn't an absolute guide to a healthy weight. When I had my first weigh-in, I weighed 512 pounds; and I had a BMI of 56.

At my ideal weight of 256, my BMI is 29. My gastric surgeon told me that he believes this is my ideal weight. He believes it's a healthy number that I can and should be able to maintain from now on. Still, that number is at the top edge of *normal* on the scale. This would tell some people that while they are doing well, they still have a long way to go. For me it means I'm in the best health of my life.

Could I do better? Sure, I can. Everyone can always do better! But it's a big step to decide to be happy with your body. I'm never going to be one of those ripped model types. But I am so much better than I used to be.

Now, women see my photo and call me handsome, sexy, and even hot. Of course, they don't see me with my clothes off. (Wink, wink!)

This is why, even though I am very happy with my body, I am currently seeking other means of exercise that will help me tone the body I do have. Because I don't have reliable transportation or a family member who can take me to a gym every day, there aren't a lot of options, but I would love to take up yoga, ballroom dancing, or maybe even martial arts. I hear there are places that now teach the visually impaired.

When you get on the scale, don't let the number ruin your day. If seeing the number on the scale (or hearing it) motivates you to do better each day, that's a good thing. If you only feel good about yourself or your day when you lose weight, then by all means stop weighing yourself so much!

This may sound like a drastic measure, but you might even consider throwing your scale away. Or hide it. Or throw out the batteries.

If you only weigh yourself when you see your doctor or when you happen to be somewhere that has a scale, it may be much healthier for you. If nothing else, it may make it far easier for you to keep yourself motivated. Remember that weighing every day isn't a good practice. It may be an ingrained habit, but you need to break it.

Think about what we tell and teach our children about keeping score in sports. There are a lot of Little League sports groups that don't keep score until after a certain age. They believe that the kids will play harder and have more fun if they don't worry about the score. They also believe the kids will focus more on building friendships this way.

I encourage you to focus on the process and on doing the right things every day than focusing on that number you see every morning. I've heard golfers say: *Don't look at the score card; just play the hole that is in front of you.*

And we've all heard the one about running your own race. I firmly believe you can accomplish your weight loss goals with or without a scale and daily weigh-ins. I believe this especially if your goal is to get to a healthy maintainable weight that will result in your living a long healthy life.

So, don't be afraid of your scale. Learn to use it as the tool it was meant to be... once a week!

Create One New Habit at a Time

When I went to my first class at TLC (Texas Laparoscopic Consultants), the instructor told us that we would have to make a lot of changes in our lives if we wanted to be successful at both losing the weight we wanted and keeping it off.

She said we would have to do things like get regular exercise, drink more water, reduce portion sizes, take vitamin supplements, get more rest, eat more protein, cut back on milk and juice, and reduce or eliminate alcohol, tobacco, and caffeine. But she went on to say not to worry because they were going to help us make these changes, and she said the best way to do so was to start with just one of them.

I learned from her that most experts believe anyone can add one habit to their life every thirty days. Basically, the idea is to make one change and stick to it for a month. Then when that month is over, you can add another new habit to your life. As time goes by these combined habits will evolve into a new healthier lifestyle.

I had already been exercising, but not as often or for as long as I should be. I had been

101

drinking more water than most people that were in the class with me prior to being told it was something to work on. I had switched to decaf tea, coffee, and diet sodas years before.

I have never smoked, and I rarely drink alcohol. I didn't do the cooking, so portion sizes were not really within my control. The vitamins I was told to take turned out to be chewable and come in a lot of great flavors, so that really wasn't a problem.

Getting more protein would turn out to be more difficult than I expected, but this was mainly because I ended up having a newer procedure called a duodenal switch that required me to get between eighty and ninety grams of protein every day.

The hardest thing for me was cutting back or eliminating milk and juice. I was raised to believe that milk and juice were good for you. You may have been raised the same way, always being told you to drink your milk so you could grow up to be big and strong.

We've all seen the ads touting the health benefits of both. There are a lot of important vitamins and minerals in both milk and juice, critical to young people whose bodies are still developing. However, as we get older and start to worry about our waistlines, we start looking for places where we can cut back.

These two beverage categories are a real problem area for a lot of people, for several reasons.

First, you can take in and process a lot more calories from liquids than you can from solids. Secondly, there are a lot of natural sugars in both. Finally, these beverages can give us comfort.

I know I didn't used to think anything about having a glass of milk before going to bed, and I'm sure you know a lot of people who couldn't imagine having breakfast without a big glass of orange juice or milk—or both. The same applies to chocolate milk. My dad got us all into drinking chocolate milk. Changing this habit was not only one of my biggest hurdles, but it was always my biggest weakness when trying to lose weight. I didn't think I would be able to manage it.

But there is a way! I don't know why it never occurred to me before, but then that's why you go to school and take classes. You do it because you need to learn from people who know more about the subject than you do. I have said before that depriving yourself doesn't work. It can work for short periods, but eventually you will get tired of not having your favorite food or drink and go back to your old ways.

So, if deprivation doesn't work, then what does? Simple—you replace your liquids with solids.

When it comes to juice there are two options. One, drink V-8 or tomato juice. Vegetable juice has less natural sugar in it than fruit does. You could also try getting a juicer and drinking celery or carrot juice that you make yourself. I prefer tomato juice made with a scoop of protein powder. This way, I get some extra protein along with a healthy drink.

The second option is to eat fruit in its raw form. You can also eat canned fruit or fruit cups, but be sure to check how they were packed. You want them in water or natural juice. You absolutely *don't* want them made or packed in any kind of syrup!

You can also now buy pre-made, sugar-free Jell-O cups with fruit inside them. Then there are applesauce and other processed fruits, but these, again, can be made with a lot of sugar, so you have to be careful. Finally, you can opt to eat freeze-dried fruit like raisins, Craisins (cranberry-raisins), blueberries, mixed fruit, etc. Just be sure to get freeze-dried fruits, otherwise you will be taking a chance on getting unnecessary sugars there, too.

As for milk, you have several options. If you can't cut back or reduce, then at least start by switching to a lower fat milk, or even a soy-based milk. There are 25 calories per cup in Silk's Almond Milk or Cashew Milk, whereas there are 250 calories in one cup of 2% milk!

The best thing would be to replace your glass of milk with low-fat cheese, string cheese, cottage cheese, etc.

You can also use yogurt. Yogurt is great because not only are you replacing liquids with solids, but you are getting a lot of protein, too. There are also enzymes in yogurt that improve the health of your digestive tract.

Because we are discussing making better food choices, it's a good time to talk about ice cream. I have replaced my ice cream with sherbet, ice milk, or frozen yogurt. There are a lot of flavors of these products to choose from. I even found a new, low-calorie dip in our grocery store that was made using yogurt. It was very tangy and went well with my allotment of twenty nacho chips.

Some other food changes my family has made is the swapping of white bread, buns, crackers, and pasta for whole wheat options. I also toast all my bread because it makes it easier for the digestive system to process it. We have replaced white rice with brown rice.

We have swapped the traditional cream gravy for a brown gravy out of a box that has nothing in it but a chemical color and flavor.

We stopped buying pre-made, frozen items like meat balls, egg rolls, and pizza rolls. We also switched to skim milk to use in our cereal. We buy plain oatmeal and grits instead of the flavored kind. We no longer deep-fry anything and we don't bread food before baking it. We don't cook eggs in bacon grease any more. We use a spray or a fake butter. We don't even use sugar in our tea and, as southerners at heart, that one was hard! When we have hamburgers, we use the 90 percent lean meat and drain off whatever grease comes out.

When we occasionally have fries, they are baked in the oven. Unlike the old days, they aren't covered in chili, cheese, or sour cream. I'm sure there are other swaps we have made and even more you can think of.

You just have to start thinking how you can make better choices… today.

What is your worst food or drink issue? Does my sharing these options give you any ideas on how you might come up with some choices that will allow you to lose weight and keep it off—without feeling deprived?

The next change I made that you can also make is to the portion sizes. When I think about the quantities of food I used to eat, I wonder why I *only* weighed 512 pounds! I was eating two or three helpings from a large dinner plate. I often had snacks and ate junk food on top of this. One of the things that got much easier after surgery was adjusting my portion sizes.

The longer we have been doing something, the less likely we are to change it. But it can be done! One of my problem areas was eating at night. When your family cooks enough food that there are leftovers, then there is plenty to choose from should you be hungry from nerves or boredom later. So, switching to smaller portions is not only about the meal, but it's also about the leftovers.

Many people feel like they almost have to have food to put away for lunch tomorrow or for a meal later in the week. Some people will feel really uncomfortable with the idea of cooking just what you need rather than what you have always prepared.

Another way you can cut down on portion sizes is in the variety. This is especially true with family meals like for Thanksgiving and Christmas. Our family meal has been shrunk down to turkey, dressing, green beans, potato salad, Watergate salad, and a Southern dish called macaroni pie. If we have dessert, there will be one pumpkin pie. By changing the menu, this means we all have to agree on what to have. Changing the diet for an entire household starts with having an honest but loving discussion about what is healthy and what you can realistically accomplish at this time.

Another way to adjust to reducing portion sizes is to change the size of your dinnerware. The plate I eat off of now is much smaller than my former one, and I use smaller bowls now, too. You can also reduce the portion of your beverages. Have you ever really looked at or thought about the sizes of the drinks that restaurants, coffee shops, and convenience stores sell? They are huge! They do this because we are always asking for more or cheaper prices or both.

More often than not a drink container or cup purchased at a convenience store won't even fit in the cup holders in our vehicles.

So, do you buy that big cup because you need it, or do you drink it because you have bought it? When Coca Cola was first sold in bottles or cans, the containers held eight ounces. Now, a common To-Go cup may hold 44, which is almost six times as much!

The thing to do is to opt for a smaller beverage. You can also drink a glass or two of water before consuming your favourite beverage and/or meal. This will help you feel fuller longer, too. I know eating smaller portions isn't easy. But I also know there are always opportunities for you to make changes in your diet if you approach things with a good frame of mind.

Small action steps to take to create new habits where your food choices are concerned are as follows:
1. Remind yourself that you are working hard to be healthy.
2. Start paying attention to leftovers and use this as a way to buy and prepare less food.

3. Buy a smaller size of plates and cups.
4. Review your recipes to see what ingredients can be replaced.
5. Increase your water intake. (I'll talk more about this shortly.)
6. Talk to your family members and ask them to contribute ideas to make your new changes less difficult on you and the whole family.

Taking vitamin supplements might also be something you need to do in your quest to create new habits. Before starting to take any supplements, however, speak with a doctor and find out what you should take.

Have you considered how much your diet may be lacking in vitamins, due to the high levels of processed foods you routinely consume?

I had to accept that I would be taking vitamin supplements for the rest of my life. I have managed this change by finding variety in the flavors available. I take iron because my modified digestive system doesn't produce enough of it, post-surgery. I take sixty milligrams a day, and my vitamins come in a tasty tropical flavor.

Iron is used in our blood to transfer oxygen throughout the body. This means if you are feeling tired and run-down, it could be from a lack of iron. This is something your doctor can easily test for should you take the time to share with them how you are feeling.

I had to have what is called *an iron panel* done. This not only lets you know your basic iron levels but more detailed information on how it is being absorbed and used in your body (or not used).

In addition to an iron supplement, I take a special multi-vitamin that has been designed to be digestible by my smaller stomach. I also take a combination of calcium and Vitamin D. The calcium is to replace vitamins normally processed from dairy that my body doesn't absorb as efficiently any more. The Vitamin D is to replace the beneficial effects of sunlight. These supplements come in many flavors including chocolate, caramel, peanut butter, and berry. With so many people working indoors under harsh florescent lights and in front of computer screens or television monitors, many people are now suffering deficiencies. I should mention that I buy all my supplements through Bariatric Advantage products via the e-store on the TLC (Texas Laparoscopic Consultants) website. However, you can buy a version of what I take over the counter now. Sometimes, I use them myself when circumstances don't allow me to have the preferred brand on hand. There are studies that prove a lack of Vitamin D or calcium can have an adverse impact on your food choices and your ability to get the best results out of your weight loss efforts.

The time that you take your vitamins matters, too. Many vitamins and minerals are lost if you take them with coffee, tea, or another caffeinated beverage. Calcium can bind with iron or other vitamins and not be properly absorbed.

I now have a schedule that starts with iron first, then multi-vitamin two hours after that, then my calcium a few hours after that. If you are going to take supplements hoping to improve your health, then it's important to take them in a method that gives you the most results for your investment.

Your doctor can do some basic bloodwork to determine what your vitamin and mineral levels are and advise you on the proper supplements to correct any existing health problems, but you have to be willing to have a real conversation with your doctor for this to happen. If you don't have a doctor you feel you can tell everything to, then either change your relationship with him or her or change doctors!

Next up in in the creation of new habits is to address your sleep issues, if you have any, and change them.

I needed to get more rest and quality sleep. The doctors didn't have to preach to me on this one. Having been diagnosed with sleep apnea and having to sleep with a CPAP machine, I know the value of getting quality rest. This not only applies to your night-time sleep, but to those times during the day taken for real relaxation.

I didn't have a real problem with this. No matter how hard I would be working to build my businesses, I knew I had to get sleep. I knew and still appreciate the value of taking time during the day to put down the laptop and turn off my smart phone to just enjoy a good book, movie, TV show, conversation, meal, etc. **I know you might think that you don't have enough time to sleep, much less rest, but both are essential for proper body functions! Both are needed to repair and rejuvenate the body and mind.**

I challenge you to try getting at least eight hours of sleep each night for a week and see what it does for not only your energy levels but your concentration levels. Studies have proven that sleep-deprived people make even worse food decisions than those who get enough sleep. Think about the diet of an average college student. Could you survive on that now? Would you want to? Can you honestly see yourself losing weight and keeping it off living on a few hours' sleep bolstered by caffeine or energy drinks?

To get a better rest, some pointers include removing light and noise from your bedroom, choosing a new bed or linens that make you as comfortable as possible, add soothing sounds and aromas to your environment, and practicing meditation or having some quiet time to put all the day's troubles out of your mind before putting your head on the pillow. Turn off all your electronics, too, if you can. You would be surprised how hard it is to sleep when they make a noise that sounds like something you think is important.

I'll give you one example from my own life. I now turn off the email program on my laptop before going to bed. (I don't turn the computer off because, with my Mac, it isn't required, and I use it so much during the day and even sometimes at night that I don't like shutting it down.) But that ding my mail program makes when I have new mail disturbs me. I have clients all over the world and sometimes they email me during normal business hours that happen to be the middle

114

of the night where I am, depending on what time zone they are in. Those dings no longer bother me since I started closing that email program!

Not getting a sufficient amount of sleep also has definite health risks, including high blood pressure, increased stroke risk, impotence, a general lack of interest, and increased risk of depression. If you make improving your sleep time a part of your new healthier lifestyle, you will be much better off for it!

Now, as promised, let's talk about your water intake.

I mentioned earlier that I was always a big water drinker. But even then, I wasn't drinking enough water. And I was drinking a lot of coffee and soda that were forcing that water right back out of my system. Now, I drink four to five plastic water bottles every day. It may sound like a lot, but it's really not, and I've gotten used to it. Of course, it helps that there are so many low-calorie, flavored mixers to add to the water. You can add lemon to your plain water. You can also make it seem better by drinking it in small amounts.

Also, it's much more socially acceptable now to drink water and carry your own water bottle with you everywhere you go. It's a lot easier to envision yourself drinking a cup of water than it is imagining yourself drinking several large bottles a day. White tea and green tea both have a lot of health benefits, so drinking your water in the form of tea can be done, too.

Even switching to decaf coffee can be a big step forward. If you think you need the real stuff first thing in the morning, then try switching your afternoon or mid-day cup for a cup of decaf, tea, or a glass of water. And just to remind you, don't forget to consider drinking smaller cups!

The changes you make and the habits you create are more about what you can do instead of what you can't or haven't managed yet. Remember, it's all a process!

I told you at the beginning of this chapter that I didn't get where I am overnight. I wasn't even sure I could make all these changes. But I believed in my teachers and did it one new habit at a time, just like I'm telling you how to do it.

So, get up every day and congratulate yourself for the changes you have managed to make *and maintain*, and then challenge yourself to add just one more.

Before I finish this chapter, I want to talk briefly about satisfaction or satiation. While this next one wasn't on the list of changes I was told to make, I think it's important to discuss.

I had to learn how to feel satisfied and full with the amount of food I am now consuming. If you ever have had times where you have eaten a full meal and then found yourself hungry fifteen minutes or an hour later, you'll know that this is an important topic. I know there are the jokes surrounding Chinese food, that you're hungry a half-hour later after eating it. But feeling that urge to eat more can happen after consuming *any meal*.

There are some definite tricks you can use to keep this from happening. First, you shouldn't drink while eating. I was told that if you wait at least fifteen minutes after eating before taking a drink of anything that you will feel fuller longer. Next, never eat while standing up, driving, or performing other tasks. Also, you shouldn't be watching TV, listening to music, or reading while eating. You want to sit in a comfortable chair, but it's better to sit at an actual table.

Your goal is to make eating an enjoyable experience. To do this, do the following:

1. Eat a table.
2. Eat off smaller plates or out of smaller bowls.
3. Eat slower, and concentrate on chewing your food.
4. Use a smaller fork or spoon to eat.
5. Put your fork or spoon down in between bites.
6. Savor your food.
7. Pay attention to the textures and aromas of your food.
8. Concentrate on enjoying your experience and appreciate that you have food to eat.
9. Make eating a ritual you look forward to.

Have you ever seen someone at a restaurant that has ordered a fine bottle of wine? There is a whole procedure of opening the bottle, sniffing the cork, pouring a small amount to taste, swirling the wine, and sniffing the wine, before eventually drinking it.

We want to make each meal like drinking a fine wine. If this means that you have to put out actual china and silverware to remind you to really enjoy the meal, then do it! What is all that fancy dinnerware for if no one is going to enjoy it? If this will help you lose weight, then all the better!

Some people talk about changing the color of your dishes. For obvious reasons, I wouldn't know if that works or not. If you feel like it helps you to eat off of blue plates and hanging purple wallpaper in your eating area, then do it!

I believe that using a smaller fork or spoon can be a big help in appreciating your food and will lead to a higher level of satisfaction, what the experts call *satiation*.

While I have no scientific research to point to, I honestly believe that dousing your food in a lot of salt, pepper, ketchup, relish, mustard, or other condiments or spices is not at all helpful to being satisfied. I think this is because by having to add so much to the food you are almost saying to yourself that you won't enjoy it. I haven't added salt to food in over thirty years. I started in college when I realized that putting a bunch of salt on campus food wasn't going to make it all that much better.

If there are certain foods that you really enjoy, I advise you to include them more often in your meal plans. For example, I love mushrooms, onions, and black olives. I can eat them on just about anything, including eggs! I also enjoy spicy foods. I have even bought Monterey Jack string cheese because I feel better after eating it than I do after eating cheddar or some other cheese.

One other thing about making your eating experience enjoyable is to allow yourself to have a period of relaxation and digestion once you are finished eating.

Don't jump up to go do something right away. Those dishes can wait. None of your other chores will get angry at you if you are a few minutes late! Instead, have a conversation with someone. Or sit quietly and read.

The goal here is to make your food and the experience of eating it as enjoyable and satisfying as possible. By doing this you are far less likely to be hungry as often. You may still have those times when you eat and shouldn't be hungry, but are.

We all do. We eat out of fear, anger, fatigue, or because we don't have anything else to do. No one wins all the time. But enjoying your meal is a change you can make that will help you cut down on these times.

So, what new habit will you start today?
Start with something easy, something that will make you feel good when you accomplish it. Do that one small thing for a

month and then pick something else to add to it the next month.

As you continue to make progress towards living a healthy life, you should start to see more and more progress towards your weight loss goals.

Just remember that having one bad day doesn't mean you are a failure. **Failure only comes when you quit trying.**

Most people only get tempted to quit when they are hurtful to themselves with their own thoughts and words. Remember to practice your positive self-talk and affirmations, and to take one step at a time.

When things do work out and you feel great about your progress, be sure to celebrate your wins.

This can be a problem area for people who have been trying unsuccessfully to lose weight, because how you celebrate your victory, if not by eating?

There are many things you can do to celebrate. Here are some of my own.
One, I post photos or share my wins on social media. I do this with humility so people love them. I routinely get my most likes and

comments from personal posts about milestones reached.

Two, I take time away from work and do something fun. I may watch a movie, listen to a good audio book, go for a swim, take a walk, enjoy a bubble bath, or have a great cup of coffee. Take some time and play Words with Friends, Jeopardy, or Trivia Crack online.

Three, call up your best friend and tell them the news.

Four, go shopping and buy something new, or just go and look around. Just make sure that the purchase or time spent looking is in accordance with the level of your current accomplishment!

Five, take a road trip or go on a vacation.
Six, take some new photos of yourself. (This is one I need to do more of!) You can also make videos!

Be as creative about your rewards as you were with the steps you took to lose weight.

I am sure you will come up with some rewards on your own, too, using these ideas to get you started. It's my hope that this book will put you in the right frame of mind for finding creative solutions to long-standing problems in your life, whether they are professional, personal, or physical.

I'm looking forward to hearing your success stories (and having people tell me about or describe your amazing new photos and videos to me). I hope you will share your progress on Facebook and Twitter.

I also hope this book is what you needed to help you succeed with losing weight and becoming the person you were meant to be!

To Be Social or Anti-Social?

Many overweight people tend to stay home instead of going out and attending events. It is much better for our psychological health for us to be social, however, instead of being anti-social and living like a hermit.

In this chapter, I will give you some pointers on how to prepare yourself for when you *do* go out. I will also let you know when it's okay to stay home.

In the spring and summer, many people have barbecues and neighborhood parties. Most people struggle with how to maintain their healthy lifestyle without just saying NO every time the phone rings from someone asking them to come to an event.

There are many things you can do, but a lot of your choices depend on how far along you are in your process. Attending parties where the main focus will be on food is harder on people who have just started making changes than it is on someone whose eating habits are far more practiced and ingrained.

So, let's look at what you can do.

First, decide whether or not you want to go to the event. We all know there are some people who just rub us the wrong way. We know they will push our buttons and cause us to eat recklessly.

Consider whether or not there will be drinking or smoking at the event. Can you deal with people drinking beer or alcoholic drinks without it being a trigger for you to binge? Can you handle people smoking cigarettes, cigars, or pipes without wanting to distract yourself with food? If you can, then, by all means, attend the event. If not, it may be best to decline the invitation.

It is better for your well-being to decline an invitation than it is to go to an event and spend time with people who don't have your best interests at heart.

There are times in our lives when we are more vulnerable to over-eating. You may already be in the wrong frame of mind to be around piles of food. If this is the case, there is nothing wrong with just staying home. Remember, this is about *you* and *your* success.

But what if the event is a party you can't get out of attending? Here, I am thinking of office parties, weddings, funerals, or church pot-luck dinners. In these cases, you have to have a strategy in place and take some preventative steps before you even leave the house.

One thing you must do is drink plenty of water. Water is one of those things that does a lot of healthy stuff for you. It hydrates your body and can make your skin look and feel better. It can even help with your ability to handle stress as being dehydrated can lead to an overall ill feeling. In this case, it will fill you up and make you less hungry at the event.

Another thing to do is to get plenty of sleep the night before the event. You should be getting plenty of quality rest on a regular basis, anyhow, to maintain your good health, but if you aren't getting eight hours of sleep every night, you should at least make it a point of getting it the night before a big party. Well-rested people make better food choices. It is also important not to skip your exercise routine on the day of the event because you are rushing to get ready for your big night. That fifteen or thirty minutes will help you stay in a good frame of mind and keep you feeling positive. At least, this has been my experience! Prior to leaving the house, you should also have a small, high-protein snack. In addition to water, protein also takes up space in your tummy and makes it easier to say no to all that food. In addition, you should consider taking a snack or a water bottle with you. This used to be something only a really dedicated health nut would do, but thankfully things have changed, and carrying a water bottle wherever you go has become much more acceptable.

If the event is one where everyone brings a dish, you should bring a healthy one (or consider bringing two dishes—one for everyone else, and one for you and the other people who will want a healthy food option).

Remember, too, that there is no rule that says you have to stay for the entire event. Stay for fifteen minutes, meet your obligation, and then leave. If you bring a dish, then put it in a container you won't miss, such as a disposable pan or plastic container, because you might have to leave it there. When you leave, tell someone you have to go but they can have the dish or return it to you later. No Tupperware container is worth ruining your new food habits over! You likely won't be the only one there who is concerned about their weight and their health. Perhaps others have decided to give themselves a pass for the day. Perhaps they have decided to do the more destructive thing and say to themselves that, no matter what, they are going to be fat, so why worry about it?

It's usually after a few bites of something that you know you shouldn't have that people decide to say *the heck with it* and go on a binge. There is nothing wrong with eating a few bites of something you wouldn't ordinarily have, as long as you don't let it affect your mood and your attitude about yourself. Making excuses, however, is not how you should approach things!

Also, just because it is a party, nothing says you have to eat the whole slice of cake, pie, or sweetbread that someone says you just have to try. You can allow yourself a small slice, but you don't have to eat all of it. You can also refuse it altogether.

If you can, fill your own plate with good food choices.

It's easier for you to maintain your diet if you fill your own plate than it is when you have others bring you a loaded plate… *which they will do!* People will do this even when they know you are trying hard to lose weight. Some of them do it because they don't know any better. They have always shown love by offering full plates and it's the only way they know to act. Others will be jealous of your desire and ability to change your habit's and improve your health. These people are the ones to avoid. I have been at family dinners where I have had to hold on to my plate so someone didn't try to give me more food. It can get a bit irritating to have to keep saying, "No, thank you, I'm full," or "No, thank you, I don't want any of that." But you can do it!

During the party, it is good to socialize. Talking with others is expected, and you should seek out these positive experiences! I have found that, since having my gastric surgery and losing the weight, I will meet at least one person who wants to talk to me. They want to know about my progress and what was involved. They ask about what I'm doing in my business and personal life. It's great to be able to share things about myself with those who are genuinely interested! You can reciprocate the conversation by asking them questions about their life and their family. Even if you are usually shy or introverted, there will be opportunities for one-on-one conversations that aren't there when your focus is on food.

Another thing that can help at these events is having activities to distract you from the available food. It's best if people have games planned for during the meet-up. I don't play Texas Hold 'Em poker, but a lot of my family members do, and this practice of playing cards has become a part of our family gatherings. However, I like playing Rummy and regular poker, and so I sometimes take my deck of Braille cards with me.

About a year ago, I bought an iPhone, so I now have a phone that's like a little computer. If I get really stuck for a distraction, I can play Trivia Crack or listen to sports on it. I can even surf the net and reply to my emails.

Since most of my family is in the amusement industry, I can often talk some business at these family dinners. I may hear that one of my cousins is looking to buy or sell something. Someone else may ask if I had any hits on an item they have listed, or any ideas how to make it more appealing. The point is, there are a lot of things you can do to distract yourself and others from the food. At an Oscar party, you can guess on who will win what and keep track. The conversation about the winners and how well you are doing can be great to keep you from thinking about food. The same thing can apply to filling out a bracket for the NCAA basketball tournament or making fake wagers on some of the crazy Super Bowl bets that they offer in Vegas.

Nowadays, you can often find others at just about any event who are bloggers, podcasters, writers, or speakers who you can have a conversation with and share ideas.

You have to get to the point where you aren't just going to a party for the food. If you can make that shift in your thinking, then you can find all kinds of activities, people, and other distractions to keep you from loading up and wrecking your diet.

It's important to note that these suggestions are about how to deal with social situations. I haven't covered them all, and I can't, because they are too numerous.

However, one other situation just came to mind, and that's what to do when you are out shopping. This may sound stereotypical, but men usually go shopping to buy a particular item they need, and then leave. Women shop more to find out what is available in hopes of finding something they want. Regardless of your shopping style, it's a challenge being in a store located a mall, without thinking of food, because of the fast food outlets or food courts.

I used to be part of a carnival, so I know the power that exhaust fans can have on the aromas of freshly cooked food. You need to come up with strategies to keep from eating what the vendors are trying to sell! They don't care about your success or failure with eating healthy. They only care about getting you to spend!

This is just as true when shopping for groceries as it is for any other kind of shopping. For example, how often do you find yourself buying a box or bag of whatever free snacks they offered you while at Walmart or Sam's Club?

Before you go shopping, make sure you drink your water, eat before you leave, and take a snack with you.

Now let's talk about after the party. For argument's sake, say you didn't have a good night. Say your nemesis was there, and while you wanted to show them you were a new person, you ended up eating more than you should have. Well, this is where you have to remind yourself to be kind to yourself.

You have to learn to forgive yourself and work to do better next time. You are not a bad person. You aren't a failure. You just didn't succeed that particular night, or do as well as you had hoped you would.

That's okay.

Quite often, we have to practice new attitudes and new techniques a while before they become a true habit. You don't just wake up magically one morning and no longer have food cravings… or eat too much at parties!

Even though I had surgery, there are still certain people I try not to spend a lot of time around and there are still some foods that I know I have to avoid, such as French bread, cornbread, tater tots, French fries, and Fritos. No one is perfect, not even me! The thing is, I have more good days than bad ones. So, I hope this has you motivated to become someone who can go to a party have a good time and still be able to love yourself in the morning. You can still love yourself, even if you don't love what you did.

The final thing to consider regarding parties or events is what to do if you want to host a party at your place. First of all, if you aren't up to surviving going to a friend or family member's house for a party, then you sure as heck aren't ready to host one! This is not only because of all the food you will be around before and during the event, but also because many people will leave food at your house and the leftovers can be daunting.

When food is available to you, especially in large amounts, it's hard not to find something you like. Also, there is the age-old fear about wasting good food. We can find a lot of reasons to eat if that is what we want to do. Having a mountain of the stuff in your refrigerator or on your table is a recipe for disaster.

If you do have to host a party (such as a birthday party for your child), then do your best not to prepare more food than you really need. Also, give leftovers away as quickly as possible and freeze the rest rather than putting them in the refrigerator.

Do not be disappointed with yourself if you bow to pressure from the family or tradition to make all of their favorites the way you have always made them. You can only do your best. Each time you attend a party—or host one—you will get better at it. Accept your past shortcomings and aspire to do better next time.

My dad used to tell us the Iveys aren't losers. He said, "We may not win as often as we like, but that doesn't make us losers."

He was right. At this point, you are just someone who hasn't succeeded yet. You haven't found your winning formula, but you will!

With what I have shared, combined with your creative mind, I know you can maintain a healthy diet and lifestyle. Having faith in yourself and your ability to get better every time is how you will eventually become the person you were meant to be.

You can do it as long as you continue to make small improvements and get better each day!

I believe in you, and know you can do it!

Now you just have to believe in yourself, and that's what the next chapter is about.

Believe In Yourself

In the Disney movie, Dumbo, the plucky little elephant, was told to believe in the magic feather. Through the magic of Disney, he learned he could fly.

We all have to have faith in something, even if it's just the faith that this time we will be successful.

If you don't believe in yourself, in the process, in your team, in God, in the Universe, or in *something*, it's very hard to accomplish *anything*.

As you well know, losing weight and keeping it off is one of the hardest things to achieve.

When I had my surgery, I spent six months preparing for it. I had gotten to know the surgeon and all his staff. I had been given tools to try that had worked in my real, everyday life. So I never doubted that, this time, I would make it.

I hope you can find faith in the fact that these simple techniques I am sharing with you are things *anyone* can do.

I'm not asking you to make changes that work great when life is going well but aren't practical when real life intrudes on your plans. I don't want this book to be like those makeover shows you see where the guest looks amazing after hours of being worked on by trained hairdressers and make-up artists in a style that you just know they can't maintain in a life with a job, a husband, kids, etc.

But I also hope you have faith in something else.

I've been guided and or protected many times by the power of the Holy Spirit. You may not realize it at the time but God—or the universe (whichever makes you more comfortable)—is working for your benefit.

As long as you work towards your goals with an attitude of faith and belief that you deserve to be thin and healthy, you will get there!

To prove this, I will share two examples from my own life.

When I decided to consider having gastric surgery, my doctor said she would find a clinic that would take my insurance. I live near Houston, Texas, a city that is almost driven by the medical field. However, there was only one place that would take my insurance: the Texas Laparoscopic Consultants. I mention their name again because I am truly grateful I was directed to them. I couldn't go anywhere else in the whole east half of Texas!

It turned out that they were *and are still* ranked the best in the state, with my surgeon, Dr. Terry Scarborough, being twice voted the best bariatric surgeon in the whole state.

Their interns are routinely recruited to practices in other states or countries. They have a philosophy that once you are their patient, you are part of their family for life (which I mentioned in the chapter about strengthening your support system). They insist on preparing you with information and evaluating your psychological well-being prior to the surgery. They monitor you endlessly after the procedure. It's only because of their real concern for their patients that I found out I have a disease called CLL, Chronic Lymphocytic Leukemia. Because of them, we found it very early, and my oncologist tells me that I can live a long happy life in spite of the diagnosis.

Now, we know to have my white blood cells monitored regularly, so that if further treatment is required we can do it right away.

I honestly believe I was sent to these people for a reason. I also feel as though I will be able to inspire and motivate people for many years to come.

The other experience I'd like to share has to do with my teeth.

After years of neglect, I now see a dentist regularly. They have helped correct a lot of the damage that has been done over the years. Recently, I had a terrible pain. My dentist took x-rays and said I needed to have a root canal. He checked my insurance and quoted me a price of $1400.

His business manager suggested I enroll in an additional program that would help with these costs. I did, and that brought the price down to just under $500. But $500 is not mere pocket change to me! (Do you have an extra $500 just sitting around?)

I asked them to prescribe me some painkillers while my family and I worked to raise the money. I also prayed every night for God to take away the pain in my mouth. Eventually, the pain lessened to the point where I no longer needed the pain meds. Because I have been blessed with being pain-free, there have been other priorities for that money. It may be that the tooth is healed. It may be that at some point in the future I will still have to have a root canal. But the fact that I can work, exercise, enjoy my food, and get good rest at night is all because of prayer.

I hope all this talk about faith doesn't turn you off. For those of you who believe in God, a higher power, or the universe, I hope this reminds you that even weight loss should be prayed for!

For those who don't believe in anything spiritual, I hope it doesn't cause you to disregard all the techniques and experiences I have shared with you.

Whether it's faith in God or faith in yourself, you have to believe in *something*.

They say the most successful sports teams start with great coaches. The one thing great coaches have the ability to do is to get their players to buy into their approach.

My approach is a combination of making better food choices, getting regular, moderate and repeatable exercise, praying to my God, meditating, and maintaining a positive attitude by only allowing uplifting encouraging people

and media into my life. (I'll talk about media more in the next chapter.)

There may not be anything earth-shattering in my formula, but I'm hoping that by sharing the *how* of this approach I can give you some ideas for techniques that will work in *your* particular situation.

Remember to be kind and loving towards yourself. If something works, repeat it. If something causes you to have a setback, then identify what happened, and don't allow yourself to be in the same situation again.

I hardly ever use the word *failure*. To me, the only failure comes from someone who has given up *trying*.

Don't ever stop trying!

Today could be the best day you have ever known, or it could be one of those days you choose to forget—but, either way, tomorrow you can do *better*. You just have to keep your heart and mind open to the possibilities and not beat yourself up for any past shortcomings. I have faith in you, so I hope you will decide that *this time* you believe you will succeed. I know you have it in you!

Accentuate the Positive

When I talked about strengthening your support system, I mentioned that you have to be careful who you let into your circle. I talked to you about how you need to seek out positive supportive people and eliminate those who are only going to drag you down.

The same thing applies to what you read, watch, or listen to.

Now, I'm not saying you should be perfect and only partake in things that will be good for you, but I want to encourage you to take a good, hard, and long look at *the books and magazines you read, the music you listen to, the radio shows you follow, and the movies and TV shows you watch.*

Stop and think about these things for a few minutes. Close your eyes now, and contemplate this.

Is there anything that is a regular part of your life that is causing you negative feelings? If something angers you to the point that your blood pressure rises and you can't focus on other tasks, then I would suggest you replace them with people or programs that make you feel calm or relaxed or that make you feel positive and energized. One of the things I do—that I believe more people should adopt—has to do with watching limited newscasts.

Just because there is what they call a 24-hour news cycle, it doesn't mean I have to embroil myself in the news! Unless there is some unusual event that calls for more, I watch one hour of news a day. (Okay, I don't actually watch it, because I'm blind, but I listen to it.)

I listen to the local and the national news before dinner. That's it.

The truth is that the few times when I have been at places where I had to watch more news, I didn't notice any change from the 4:00 to the 5:00 to the 6:00 to even the 10:00 or 11:00 broadcasts. I decided there are a lot of better ways I can spend my time. I also don't listen to hours of sports talk or political talk radio. I would much rather spend that time having a real conversation with someone I personally know than listen to everyone else spout off. I honestly think that more people would accomplish more just by replacing the talking heads of TV and radio with books, educational podcasts, and good music. (And when I say *good music*, I don't mean only classical or Gregorian chanting!) I listen to everything from country and blue grass to classic rock and Big Band Swing to music from symphonies and Broadway musicals. When someone I know and trust recommends it, I will also listen to some rap and heavy metal. You can find good lessons in many places!

You might be wondering about my reading library. I split it between biographies, personal development books, and a variety of fiction. My book criteria is that they tell a good story. I insist on complicated story lines, vivid setting descriptions, and complex characters who grow and develop over time.

As for television, this is a little harder because the networks conspire to put lesser shows between those we just can't miss. You have the choice of not watching, trying to find something else for a half hour, or watching a show that you don't consider a good use of your time.

I find that the longer I go on my path, the less willing I am to give these people time that they haven't earned with their best work. I have books, music, old time radio shows, graphical audio novels, movies, and different TV show episodes on my computer.

Because a lot of people eat when we are angry or nervous, it is important to cut down on those things that set us off. If listening to the latest about either political party gets you all charged up, then maybe you should cut down on the number of hours of this you listen to. Just try swapping 30 minutes or an hour of what you usually take in for something more positive. When a show comes on your TV that you know you are only watching because of the next show that comes on after it, try picking up a book or even a magazine and reading for that half hour. Focus on doing different, positive things. If there is something else in your life that you have been thinking about or dreaming about for a long time, try reading about that subject, listening to podcasts about it, or watching some YouTube videos that are helpful.

Even sports can be a problem for some people. If turning on the television to watch football, basketball, golf, tennis, soccer, auto racing, or some other sport means a day of eating junk food and drinking sodas or beer, then how about cutting back on the number of events you watch and go outside for some of that time? Start using that smart phone of yours to do something other than check scores or follow your fantasy teams!

One of my best role models in this area was my dad. He was one of the most positive people you would ever want to meet. Even in hard times, he would have a smile on his face or tell a joke to make you laugh. I can remember many times he would be watching the animal channel. He said it always made him feel better to see nature.

In today's world, the easiest place to find that is on TV or the internet. He also used to say it made no sense to him for someone who was sad to watch soap operas or other sad shows. He thought that if you wanted to be happy, you should start by watching comedies. He didn't care for those with a lot of cussing in them, but he loved the old TV shows from the "golden age of television."

Before I finish on the subject of media, I need to get metaphorical for a moment. I need to mention the images that play on the movie screen of our minds. I know far too many people who can't move forward because they are constantly replaying events from their past in their heads and beating themselves up for past failures.

We have to not only create new memories, but stop replaying all the old ones! When it comes to our own voice, we have to decide to change the channel or destroy the old videotapes and move on. It's not easy to forgive ourselves, but it's just one more area where we have to eliminate those things that drag us down or drain our energy.

We have a choice about who we let into our lives. We also have choices as to what voices we let into our hearts and minds. The more of these voices that are positive and uplifting, the higher your chances are for long-term success.

More activity and fewer triggers for eating to excess are ideal. How much of what you read, watch, and listen to are helping you move forward? How much of it is sabotaging your good intentions and hard work?

Prior to having gastric surgery, I learned to change many of my habits. It was made clear to me that lifelong success with managing my weight would only come from changing my lifestyle, which would require changing many of my attitudes about food. As I have continued to progress, I have realized that the process has also changed me. It's the continual daily action as well as learning more about myself and the reasons why more people don't lose weight and keep it off that has motivated me to write this book and share my success strategies.

You want every tool at your disposal, to have that extra advantage. You want to use every little trick you can come up with. By improving the quality of what you allow into your head, you will become more positive and responsible in other areas of your life.

The reason for my continued success is knowing what foods to eat or avoid, coupled with my commitment to improve myself.

I hope you will make the commitment to improve your body, mind, and spirit. It's only by realizing that they are all involved in successful weight loss that you are finally going to achieve your goals!

Losing weight and keeping it off is something that you will have to work on and improve every day.

As Louis Armstrong sang, "You've got to accentuate the positive, eliminate the negative, latch on to the affirmative, and don't mess with Mr. In-between."

Now, before I conclude this chapter and this book, I just want to say that I've done my best to share what I've learned during my experience with having gastric surgery and all the other changes it resulted in. While this chapter may be called the end, or the conclusion, I'm hesitant to call it that. **If I have learned anything from my journey,**

it's that you never get to a place where it is over.

There is always more thing you can do or more things you will want to guard against to maintain your good health once it's achieved.

I hope you have also learned through these lessons that achieving good health isn't a *thing* but a *process*. You and your body are a work in progress. Thanks to doctors, scientists, and fellow strugglers, there will always be more information, advice and suggestions.

Thanks to farmers, grocers, advertisers, and processed-food manufacturers, there will probably always be new tricks played upon those of us who want to get healthy and stay that way.

I have had to make many changes, most of which I wasn't sure I could manage at the time. I have had to wrap my head around the idea that I *could* and *would* be not skinny, but would be at the right weight for my height, age, and bone structure.

I never thought I would be what is called handsome or sexy, but thanks to my female friends who I know will be honest with me, this has happened. Several have even told me that when I send out emails, I should include my photo, because I sure make an impression now!

I didn't set out to be attractive to women. My goal was to avoid an early death.

At this point, I want to remind you that there are a lot of little improvements or changes you can make in your life. You just have to have the desire to make them.

If you keep your heart and mind open to new ideas and unusual solutions to your problems, you can find even more than the ones I have shared here.

I think I told you that I'm more about results than how I look doing it or what people think about me while I am. I don't need style points. The only person I am competing with is myself. So, I try new things. If they work, I repeat them. If they don't work, then I avoid doing them again.

I use all the tools I have mentioned throughout this book, such as swapping poor food choices for better ones; replacing liquids with solids; reducing or eliminating caffeine, alcohol, and tobacco; getting more regular repeatable

exercise; drinking a lot of water; taking vitamin supplements; decreasing my portion sizes; using my support network; making peace with my scale and my mirror; making my health part of my daily schedule; removing negative people and other negative influences from my life; practicing modern meditation; and, most importantly, being kind to myself and forgiving myself when the results aren't up to my expectations.

I genuinely want you to succeed. I want you to be thinner, happier, more beautiful, and sexier than you are now. I want you to replicate my success and become the person you *want* to be... the person you were *meant* to be... the person you *deserve* to be.

Whether you go from never exercising to walking for ten minutes a day, or go from exercising for five minutes to running a marathon, you need to remember to focus on the positive changes you are making.

I know how much better I feel physically, mentally, and emotionally since getting my weight under control.

I've seen my life open up to many new possibilities. I have new found confidence and more courage.

I want your family to know the person you can be.

I want your community to be blessed by someone who has more to share because you have the problem with your weight under control.

I want all of these things for you, *and more!*

You can do it. *I know you can.* Start with taking one small step… today.

Remember, it's not the cookie; it's the bag!

About the Author

Born into a family of carnival owners in Texas, USA, Maxwell Ivey lost his sight at age 12. Having a natural gusto for life, Max graduated college and became heavily involved in the Eagle Scouts.

He also worked in the family business alongside his brothers until his father succumbed to lung cancer.

Faced with his own mortality, Max made some life-altering changes.

He underwent gastric surgery and lost over 250 pounds. He started his own business, buying and selling amusement rides, and learned how to blog using software for visually-impaired people.

Overcoming many obstacles, Max made a name for himself online and now shares his experiences on The Blind Blogger.

Max's favourite things entail teaching and helping others achieve their goals and so he began another business: personal coaching.

Max now spends his days singing, reading, blogging, working, writing, creating videos, and coaching.

Max would like to travel the world one day and meet his many online friends and clients in person. He'd also like to meet a special lady to share his life with.

Maxwell Ivey can be found on social media, too, so please connect with him on:

1: Facebook at
https://www.facebook.com/Mr.Midway

2: LinkedIn at
https://www.linkedin.com/in/maxwellivey

3: Twitter using @maxwellivey or
https://twitter.com/maxwellivey

4: The Midway Marketplace at
http://midwaymarketplace.com/

To stay updated and be notified when other books are released, please visit The Blind Blogger at http://theblindblogger.net/ and sign up to Max's email list!

Be sure to pick up a copy of Max's book *Leading You Out of the Darkness into the Light* for additional motivation!

About *Leading You Out of the Darkness into the Light*

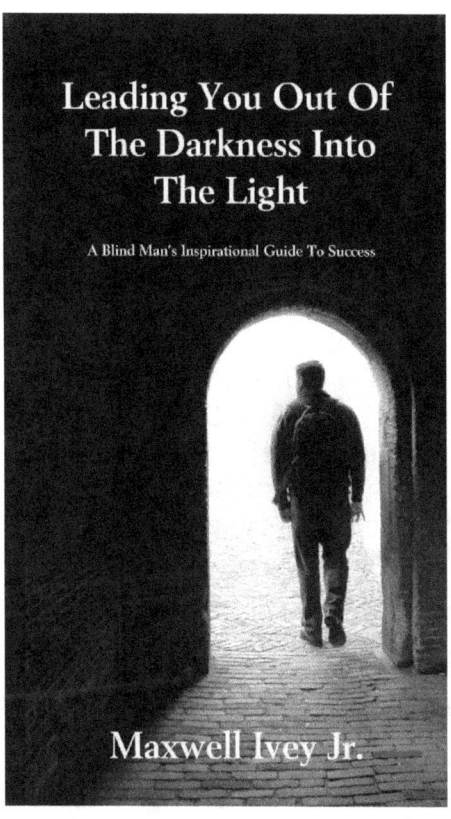

Leading You Out of the Darkness into the Light: A Blind Man's Inspirational Guide to Success is a motivational book in which Max shares the 11 steps of his success as a blind entrepreneur and the lessons he has learned from his journey.

It also provides 11 exercises for readers to do, complete with email support from the author.

It is Max's sincerest desire to help you succeed in accomplishing your goals or achieving your dreams!

Stop the excuses and get started on your success journey today!

If you purchase this book from Selz (which enables Max to earn a higher royalty percentage), you'll get 1 PDF, 11 specific steps to follow, and 11 specific, actionable exercises to complete. Purchase it via https://maxwellivey.selz.com/.

You can also purchase it in e-book or print format from Amazon.

Regardless of where you buy this book, throughout it all, Max will be with you, guiding you, helping you, and offering you his support.

This is more than just a book. *It's a chance to change your life.*

About *It's Not the Cookie, It's the Bag: An Easy-to-Follow Guide for Weight Loss Success*

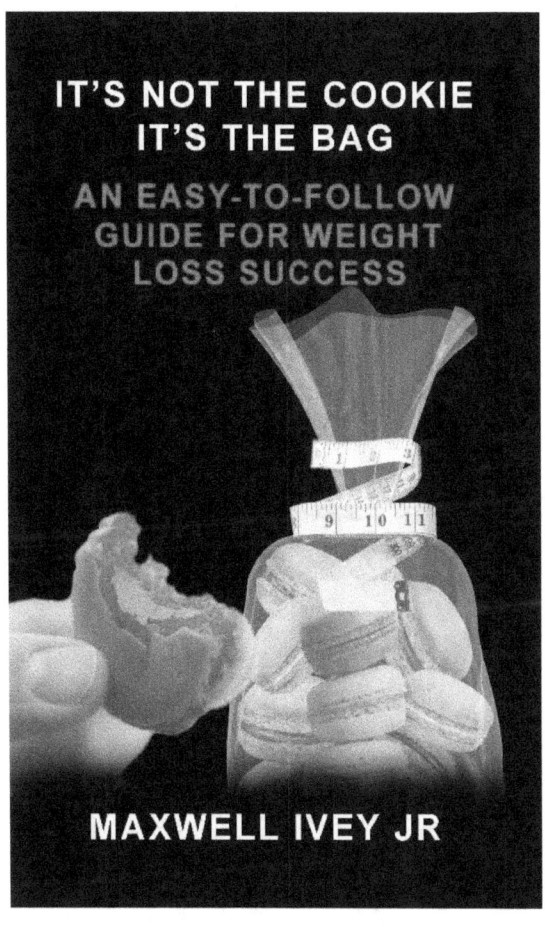

In this book, Max shared the ups and downs of his weight loss and weight maintenance journey to good health. He also revealed **the exact methods** he uses in his day-to-day life to achieve and maintain his phenomenal success. It is his hope that YOU can replicate his success and become the person you *want* to be... the person you were *meant* to be... the person you *deserve* to be... one small step at a time.

Please take the first step today.

About *The Blind Blogger's NYC Adventures (+ How You Can Make Your Dreams Come True)*

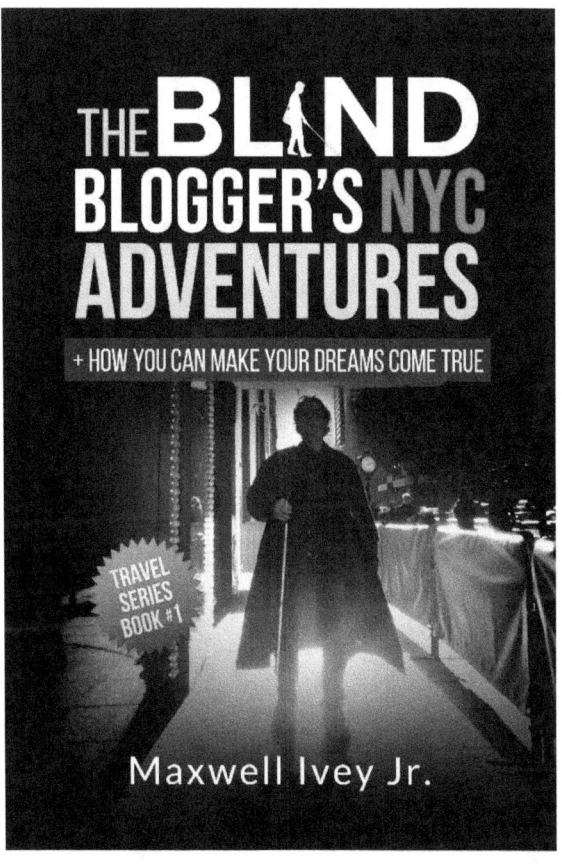

This is the first book in Max's travel series. Max has since travelled to other places, and is working on more books!

To stay updated, and be notified when other books in this series are released, please visit http://theblindblogger.net and sign up to Max's email list!

About *The Blind Blogger's First Speaking and Signing Adventures (+ How You Can Conquer Your Fears)*

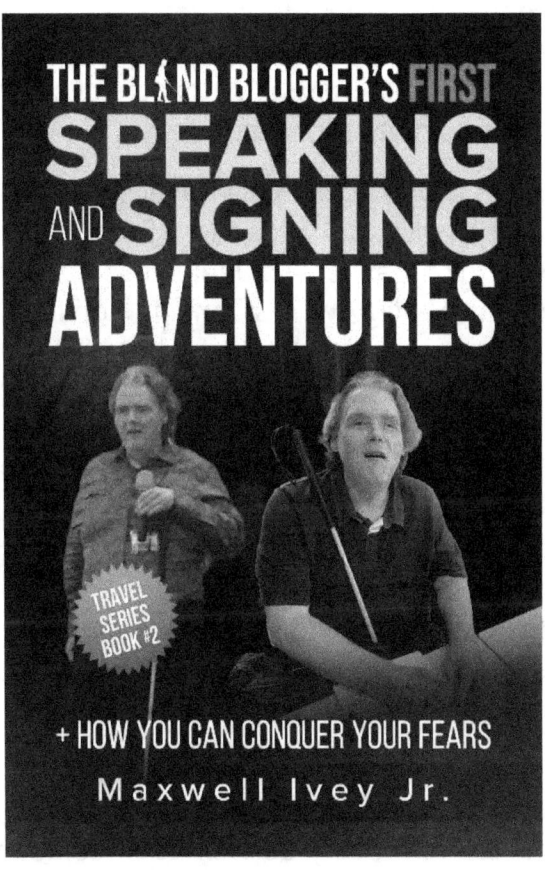

Close your eyes and imagine yourself taking a trip alone, on a tiny budget. Now, imagine taking that same trip without having sight.

Meet Max—a fearless, witty, inspiring individual who thinks nothing of traveling across the country by himself. On a limited budget, while missing trains, dealing with luggage and mobility issues, and facing unexpected circumstances, Max was determined to promote his books and become a motivational speaker.

In this second book in his travel series, Max shares wisdom gleaned from facing obstacles, teaches valuable lessons, and entertains you with stunning storytelling. Using humor and honesty, he bears his soul about the ups and downs of facing and overcoming fears and finding the positive in every situation. Commiserate with him when no one showed up at the bookstore, applaud his courage as he took the microphone and gave a powerful speech, and laugh along with him as he cracks jokes about things being so easy that even a blind guy can do them!

This book is original, entertaining, helpful, and reassuring. It's also an incredible example of bravery as well as of someone who practices what he preaches and finds solutions instead of making excuses. Use Max's advice as you challenge yourself to chase your dreams, reach your goals, face your fears, and attain new levels of success.

Above all, enjoy the ride!

This is the second book in Max's travel series. Max has since travelled to other places, and is working on more books!

To stay updated and be notified when other books in this series are released, please visit http://theblindblogger.net and sign up to Max's email list!

Upcoming Books

Max has plans for at least two more books in his travel series. To stay updated and be notified when other books in this series are released, please visit The Blind Blogger at http://theblindblogger.net and sign up to Max's email list!

www.ingramcontent.com/pod-product-compliance
Lightning Source LLC
Chambersburg PA
CBHW062207280526
45788CB00001B/480